BT/40.B/01

GROUP TREATMENTS FOR POST-TRAUMATIC STRESS DISORDER

GROUP TREATMENTS FOR POST-TRAUMATIC STRESS DISORDER

Bruce H. Young, M.S.W., L.C.S.W.
Disaster Services Coordinator
National Center for PTSD
Menlo Park, CA

Dudley D. Blake, Ph.D.
Clinical Psychologist and Co-Director
Evaluation and Brief Treatment PTSD Unit
Boise VA Medical Center
Boise, ID

USA	Publishing Office:	BRUNNER/MAZEL *A member of the Taylor & Francis Group* 325 Chestnut Street, Suite 800 Philadelphia, PA 19106 Tel: (215) 625-8900 Fax: (215) 625-2940
	Distribution Center:	BRUNNER/MAZEL *A member of the Taylor & Francis Group* 47 Runway Road, Suite G Levittown, PA 19057-4700 Tel: (215) 269-0400 Fax: (215) 269-0363
UK		BRUNNER/MAZEL *A member of the Taylor & Francis Group* 1 Gunpowder Square London EC4A 3DE Tel: 171 583 0490 Fax: 171 583 0581

GROUP TREATMENTS FOR POST-TRAUMATIC STRESS DISORDER

1 2 3 4 5 6 7 8 9 0

Printed by Braun-Brumfield, Ann Arbor, MI, 1999.

A CIP catalog record for this book is available from the British Library.
∞ The paper in this publication meets the requirements of the ANSI Standard Z39.48-1984 (Permanence of Paper)

Library of Congress Cataloging-in-Publication Data

Young, Bruce H.
    Group treatments for post-traumatic stress disorder / Bruce H.
Young, Dudley D. Blake.
        p.   cm. -- (The series in trauma and loss, ISSN 1090-9575)
    Includes bibliographical references and index.
    ISBN 0-87630-983-X (alk. paper)
    1. Post-traumatic stress disorder--Treatment. 2. Group
psychotherapy. I. Blake, Dudley D. II. Title. III. Series.
    RC552.P67Y685   1999
616.85'21--DC21   99-12798
                                                CIP

ISBN: 0-87630-983-X (case)
ISSN: 1090-9575

Dedication

For my cherished daughter Jannah and my mother Edythe Young, and in memory of my father Frank Young. For my friend Gail Lebovic, a physician for whom great love and great work are indivisible. And for my friend and music teacher, Steve Koski, whose joy revealed that all great things begin with listening.

B.H.Y.

For Alison, Emma, Sam, and Ben. The extraordinary collection of people known as my family and informal therapy group.

D.D.B.

Contents

CHAPTER 10
Group Treatment for Adult Survivors of Childhood Abuse   201

Lisa Y. Zaidi

Afterword   221

Bruce H. Young and Dudley D. Blake

Index   225

Contributors

DUDLEY D. BLAKE, Ph.D., is codirector of the Evaluation and Brief Treatment PTSD Unit at the Boise Department of Veteran Affairs Medical Center. Dr. Blake has coauthored over 30 chapters and articles. His clinical interests include PTSD assessment and treatment, cognitive therapy, and behavioral medicine.

EDWARD B. BLANCHARD, Ph.D., is the director of the Center for Stress and Anxiety Disorders at the University at Albany, State University of New York. In 1990, he was named Distinguished Professor of Psychology. Dr. Blanchard began work on PTSD at the Albany VA in 1981, focusing primarily on assessment research with Vietnam veterans. In 1990, he began collaborative research on motor vehicle accident survivors with Dr. Edward J. Hickling. Their chapter in this book is the product of that research collaboration sponsored by a grant from the National Institute for Mental Health.

DON R. CATHERALL, Ph.D., is executive director of the Phoenix Institute and an adjunct associate professor at Northwestern University Medical School. Dr. Catherall is a member of the Editorial Advisory Group of the *Journal of Traumatic Stress*, a member of the Editorial Board of the electronic journal, *TRAUMATOLOGYe*, a member of the Editorial Board of Taylor & Francis Book Series on Trauma and Loss, and author of *Back from the Brink: A Family Guide to Overcoming Traumatic Stress*.

KATHLEEN M. CHARD, Ph.D., is assistant professor of counseling psychology and director of the Center for Traumatic Stress Research at the University of Kentucky. The recipient of a National Institute of Mental Health grant, Dr. Chard is researching the effectiveness of a brief, cognitive processing therapy model for childhood sexual abuse survivors.

RAYMOND J. EMANUEL, M.D., is a member of the Center for Study of Traumatic Stress and has performed research and clinical work with a number of disaster populations including the TWA airline body recovery teams. Dr. Emanuel is a child psychiatrist with interests in family violence and child abuse.

JULIAN D. FORD, Ph.D., is director of Behavioral HealthCare Outcomes Research and associate professor in the University of Connecticut Medical School Department of Psychiatry. Dr. Ford's research and clinical interests include psychotherapy of complex PTSD, process and outcome in psychotherapy and health psychology, and trauma and disruptive behavior disorders in children.

PATRICIA A. HARNEY, Ph.D., is a clinical psychologist and research consultant at the Victims of Violence Program at The Cambridge Hospital/Harvard Medical School, where she is clinical instructor in psychology. Dr. Harney maintains a private practice in Belmont, MA.

MARY R. HARVEY, Ph.D., is a psychologist and the director of the Victims of Violence Program at The Cambridge Hospital/Harvard Medical School, where she is assistant clinical professor in psychology. Dr. Harvey maintains a private practice in Cambridge, MA.

EDWARD J. HICKLING, Ph.D., is an assistant professor in the Department of Health and Rehabilitation Sciences at Russell Sage College in Troy, NY. Dr. Hickling's earlier research in PTSD included the assessment and treatment of Vietnam veterans. Since 1990, he has collaborated with Dr. Edward B. Blanchard on psychological assessment and treatment of motor vehicle accident survivors.

ANDREW W. MEISLER, Ph.D., is a clinical psychologist at the National Center for PTSD Neuroscience Division at VA Connecticut Health Care System in West Haven, CT and is clinical assistant professor of psychiatry at Yale University School of Medicine. Dr. Meisler served as director of the Substance Use PTSD Team at West Haven from 1993 to 1998 and continues actively in clinical work and research with this population.

PATRICIA A. RESICK, Ph.D., is a professor of psychology and director of the Center for Trauma Recovery at the University of Missouri–St. Louis. Her research has focused on assessment and treatment of victims of crime with an emphasis on post-traumatic stress disorder and depression in rape victims. Dr. Resick has received several grants from the National Institute of Mental Health and National Institute of Justice.

JOSEF I. RUZEK, Ph.D., is associate director for education at the National Center for Post-Traumatic Stress Disorder. Based at the VA Palo Alto Health Care System in Palo Alto, CA. He is actively involved in providing training and support services for VA specialized PTSD program staff and other healthcare providers. Dr. Ruzek is an editor of the Guilford text *Cognitive-Behavioral Therapies for Trauma*, and his current interests include PTSD and injury in the medical setting and the interaction of PTSD and substance use.

E. K. RYNEARSON, M.D., is a clinical professor of psychiatry at the University of Washington and works in the section of psychiatry and psychology, Virginia Mason Medical Center, Seattle, WA.

CINDI S. SINNEMA, B.A., works at Separation and Loss Services, Virginia Mason Medical Center, Seattle, WA.

JUDITH STEWART, Ph.D., M.P.H., is currently the network administrator for the John D. and Catherine T. MacArthur Foundation Research Network on Socioeconomic Status and Health at the University of California, San Francisco. Dr. Stewart was previously on the staff of the National Center for PTSD and was one of the primary developers of the first PTSD inpatient treatment program for women veterans. She continues to explore the impact of a variety of stressors on mental and physical health.

ROBERT J. URSANO, M.D., is professor and chairman of the Department of Psychiatry, and professor of Neuroscience, Uniformed Services University of the Health Sciences. Dr. Ursano is the chairman of the American Psychiatric Association's Committee on Psychiatric Aspects of Disaster and has authored numerous publications on trauma and disaster. He is also director of the Center for the Study of Traumatic Stress in the Department of Psychiatry, USUHS.

JANICE J. WERTZ is a doctoral student in counseling psychology at the University of Kentucky. In addition to running cognitive processing therapy groups at the Center for Traumatic Stress Research, she is currently working on a research project examining therapist stress and burnout.

BRUCE H. YOUNG, L.C.S.W., is disaster services coordinator for the National Center for PTSD and editor of the *NC-PTSD Clinical Quarterly*. Mr. Young has been a disaster mental health consultant to the Federal Emergency Management Agency, U.S. Public Health Service, Center for Mental Health Services, National Institute of Mental Health, Department of Defense, and state departments of mental health following numerous natural and human-made disasters. He has produced and directed several educational videos, including *Children and Trauma*, winner of the 1993 National Educational Film and Video Award.

LISA Y. ZAIDI, Ph.D., is an assistant professor at Seattle University, where she teaches group dynamics, counseling, dramatherapy, and other clinical courses. Dr. Zaidi also maintains a private practice in the greater Seattle area where she specializes in individual and group therapy with adolescents and their families. She has published a number of papers on the assessment and treatment of childhood abuse and post-traumatic stress disorder and is currently writing a book based on her most recent research project, a study of community role models of effective parenting.

Preface

Trauma is ubiquitous. Nearly every adult today can recall a past event in which he or she felt endangered or felt that the lives and physical integrity of significant others was jeopardized. Whether involved as survivors or helpers, in these events, many may become overwhelmed with a sense of helplessness, terror, horror, or isolation. These reactions often persist or manifest themselves in related or delayed forms, or both. For some individuals, they can live on for months, years, or decades. Without help for these individuals in some form of psychotherapeutic treatment, their level of pre-trauma functioning may never be regained.

Group therapy[1] is among the most common modes of psychotherapy treatment for trauma survivors. Several reasons underlie this phenomenon and support the use of group treatment for this population. First, group therapy is cost efficient. Utilizing one or two therapists to provide treatment to three or more individuals costs less, in time and energy, than equal amounts of individual treatment. This advantage is particularly important in treatments that rely on information dissemination and exchange. Exposure to trauma often leads to a predictable course of signs and symptoms, and factors related to its exacerbation and amelioration can be readily presented (e.g., the therapeutic use of trauma disclosure, applied coping skills, the value of social supports, and the harmful use of avoidance via substance abuse, anger expression, and so on). The second reason that group treatment is so common is that it allows the clinician to assemble a group of survivors who have had similar trauma experiences. The shared characteristic of having survived a similar event serves as the foundation and context to promote a sense of belonging and acceptance among survivors, enables them to the recognize the universality of post-traumatic symptoms, and engenders interpersonal learning. The group becomes a therapeutic community from which the individual can process trauma and its aftermath. Third, the group setting provides a unique opportunity for therapists and patients alike to see and learn about the nature of trauma and the responses to

---

[1] Note to reader: The terms "group therapy," "group psychotherapy," and "group treatment" are used interchangeably throughout the book.

trauma that can occur, thus enhancing their awareness and understanding of trauma-related problems.

For this book, we have collected the writings of esteemed authorities who have expertise in group therapy with trauma survivors. In order to best reflect contemporary group trauma work, we have chosen several trauma populations that we believe represent the survivor groups most commonly treated using group therapy. These populations include sexual assault victims, war-zone veterans, adult survivors of child sexual abuse, trauma survivors associated with homicide, victim-survivors of disaster, disaster workers, individuals who concurrently suffer from PTSD and alcohol abuse, and traumatized families who can serve as the treatment focus. Because of the high incidence of motor vehicle accidents in the United States, we have also included a chapter for a population for whom it appears no apparent group work is being conducted, motor vehicle accident survivors. The chapter contributors provide a review of the published literature in their respective areas and have attempted to outline the structure and content of their group treatments. In addition, the contributors describe what they have found to be useful indicators and counterindicants for effective group treatment within the population with whom they work.

The book begins with a contribution by Patricia Harney and Mary Harvey, who give a remarkably concise overview of group psychotherapy with trauma survivors. In this nicely written chapter, Harney and Harvey provide a summary of five well-controlled studies employing group psychotherapy to treat traumatic stress. They describe an extremely helpful *Stages by Dimension Model of Trauma Recovery* in which they assess client functioning along eight domains. Next, the authors outline guidelines for two types of groups, one primarily psychoeducational in format and the other trauma-focused in nature, which can be followed consecutively in treating trauma survivors. Finally, the authors provide a useful clinical vignette which provides the reader with an authentic sense of how group treatment can and should work.

Next, Donald Catherall describes family group treatment for trauma survivors. For many traumatized individuals, the family may be a source of support, functioning as a therapeutic recovery environment. For others, trauma-induced psychosocial impairment may adversely affect family relations and exacerbate the traumatized person's symptoms. Dr. Catherall summarizes an elegant family model for group therapy that emphasizes the impact of trauma on the family and the group and relational processes that are manifest in family PTSD work. Dr. Catherall also describes how the effects of traumatization often stir up long-standing family conflicts, how the management of shameful feelings and other emotions become central clinical issues, and how family members can resort to blaming and interpersonal distancing as they attempt to manage the effects of trauma. Finally, Dr.

Catherall provides a summary of the recovery process for working with families whose members have been exposed to trauma.

Kathleen Chard, Patricia Resick, and Janice Wertz provide a crystal clear description of their *Cognitive Processing Therapy (CPT)* used in group work with sexual assault victims. These clinical researchers describe the principles underlying their work, including the therapeutic rationale and factors to consider in assessing and selecting clients. They provide a succinct description of their 12-session CPT protocol, propose a therapeutic posture for group therapists, and outline several critical issues in delivering this highly effective treatment. This treatment is unique in comparison to the other treatments presented in this book; it does not require group members to recount aloud details of their trauma to the other members of the group. To minimize the potential for retraumatization, the exposure component involves multiple written accounts regularly reviewed by the therapists and the members themselves.

Raymond Emanual and Robert Ursano have contributed a scholarly chapter describing group interventions with disaster workers. These experts delineate the stressors associated with disaster work, present an interactional model of stress and stress mediators, and describe an intervention model that includes primary, secondary, and tertiary interventions. Their *Integrative Group Treatment (IGT)* will serve practitioners and consultants alike in efforts to mitigate the stress of disaster workers.

Julian Ford and Judith Stewart describe their group treatment conducted at the National Center for PTSD with military veterans who present with war-related PTSD. These clinical researchers review the empirical research on group therapy with combat veterans and outline principles and techniques employed in working with this population. In this chapter, Ford and Stewart provide in-depth descriptions of the therapeutic elements of their group work, including "Facing and Transmuting Terror, Rage, Guilt, and Shame," "Encountering the Unendurable," and "Giving Voice to the Unspeakable." This chapter is sure to be a valuable reference for all practitioners, particularly advanced clinicians who conduct group therapy with military veterans.

Edward Hickling and Edward Blanchard describe their work in the individual psychological treatment of survivors of motor vehicle accidents (MVA). Despite the fact that motor vehicle accidents are the most frequently experienced trauma for American males and the second for American females, there is a virtual absence of published work on group treatment in this area. Hickling and Blanchard describe their individual treatment applications, which include education, anger management and relaxation training, therapeutic exposure, and therapy homework assignments, and they show how these components might be extended to a group format. These contributors are nothing less than pioneers in the area, and their work is likely to be an invaluable reference for the treatment providers of motor vehicle accident survivors.

Andrew Meisler describes and discusses group PTSD treatment for individuals with co-occurring alcohol abuse or dependence. Dr. Meisler reviews the current epidemiological research on PTSD and gives a solid therapeutic rationale for taking an integrative approach that combines psychiatric and substance abuse treatment components for treatment with this population. He provides information about client characteristics that have prognostic significance for group work and discusses issues related to group composition and structure. Finally, Dr. Meisler gives us a detailed description of his PTSD/alcohol abuse treatment, which includes psychoeducation about PTSD and alcohol abuse, sleep hygiene, motivation enhancement, problem solving and relaxation skills, and anger management.

E.K. Rynearson and Cindy Sinnema describe supportive group therapy for treating bereaved individuals after a homicide. These authors draw from a wealth of clinical experience with trauma survivors and provide a strikingly clear multidimensional heuristic for viewing traumatic versus separation distress. This chapter makes an invaluable contribution to the published literature on a woefully underrepresented population. In an increasingly turbulent society, this chapter should become a sought-after reference for clinicians and clinical researchers.

Though there is a rapidly increasing literature addressing disaster mental health interventions (secondary interventions), few published works exist about tertiary intervention for individuals suffering from PTSD related to disaster. Bruce Young, Josef Ruzek, and Julian Ford present a cognitive-behavioral model for groups of disaster survivors for use by practitioners who help disaster victims after the emergency and early post-impact phases. They present an array of techniques and procedures including unique forms of therapeutic exposure, cognitive restructuring, relaxation training and attentional focus on significant elements of traumatic memories, and active problem-focused coping. The 15-session model described will serve as a valuable reference for many of the clinicians who work within the context of the disaster mental health crisis counseling programs of the Federal Emergency Management Agency (FEMA).

Lisa Zaidi's chapter describing her group work with adult survivors of childhood abuse closes the book. Dr. Zaidi presents the rationale for using a time-limited treatment approach integrating theoretical and, clinical concerns, while taking into account clients' perspectives. Many of her creative approaches to building group cohesiveness can be utilized within the other models presented in this book. In addition, Dr. Zaidi provides a useful framework for education about child abuse, understanding the family context, confronting memories, expressing anger, exploring obstacles to intimacy, and nonpunitive parental discipline. Dr. Zaidi concludes her chapter with an outline of eight central goals to pursue in conducting group work with adult survivors of child sexual abuse.

These chapters should have a substantial and enduring impact on the group treatment of trauma survivors. All are written by leading clinicians and clinical researchers. They are also interesting and eminently readable. Furthermore, the protocols described in each are quite reproducible for experienced clinicians and supervised trainees. This feature makes each chapter a clinical roadmap as well as a scholarly contribution. For these and other reasons, this is an exceptional guide-book and reference for conducting group therapy with trauma survivors.

Chapter 1

Group Psychotherapy: An Overview

Patricia A. Harney and Mary R. Harvey

Group therapy is regarded by many as the treatment of choice for trauma survivors. Groups restore the commonality and connection in relationships damaged by interpersonal violence (Herman, 1992; Koss & Harvey, 1992). Individuals for whom secrecy characterized their trauma learn to speak publicly about what happened (Shatzow & Herman, 1989). Groups help individuals who feel overwhelmed by their post-traumatic symptoms to make sense of their experiences and reactions. Survivors share tools for managing intolerable symptoms. Individuals who are unable to bear traumatic affect alone or with another person may be able to do so within a larger, structured network of relationships. When traumatic affect is contained in a safe and structured manner, survivors tolerate better the integration of traumatic memories and develop a wider range of feeling. Memories that provoke previously intolerable feelings are examined and understood. The survivor who creates a sense of connection with valued others learns to value herself or himself (Harvey, 1996).

Group psychotherapy offers several clinical advantages over individual psychotherapy. In groups, survivors witness each member's learning process. This format therefore encourages a sense of empowerment among group members by deemphasizing a hierarchical relationship between individual therapist and client. Groups that are co-led allow clinicians to share the experience, which helps to manage countertransference and to prevent burnout and secondary traumatic stress. While group psychotherapy has a unique role in the process of healing from traumatic exposure, this modality has other advantages as well. Group treatment is cost-effective. The high cost of treatment and lowered rate of reimbursement for mental health services increase the need to develop accessible care.

Unfortunately, the multiply traumatized individual is even less likely to gather the resources needed to obtain treatment. At the Victims of Violence Program at The Cambridge Hospital, a group treatment program has been developed that recognizes the needs of multiply traumatized and otherwise disenfranchised individuals. That program is called *Stages by Dimensions*. In the sections that follow, current models of group psychotherapy will be described. Next, the principles and techniques that underlie a *Stages by Dimensions* group treatment model will be presented. Patient selection, treatment phases, therapists' role and contradindications will be discussed.

LITERATURE REVIEW

Several models of group psychotherapy for trauma survivors have been described in the traumatic stress literature. Very few published reports have examined the efficacy of group treatment in an experimental or quasi-experimental manner. A recent PSYCHLIT search of the trauma literature revealed five published reports of group treatment efficacy that included a comparison or wait list group (see Table 1.1). These group interventions have been guided by cognitive, behavioral, interpersonal, or psychodynamic models of treatment.

Cognitive models of trauma impact suggest that a person's beliefs about the world and himself or herself are disrupted by trauma. Post-traumatic symptoms therefore arise from changes in one's expectations of threat (Resick & Schnicke, 1992). Positive changes in one's beliefs, expectations, and attributions should bring about a reduction in post-traumatic symptomatology. Behavioral models focus on the survivor's acquisition of fear and the sustained fear response that may last long after exposure to a traumatic event. Cognitive and behavioral group treatments rely on a particular set of techniques that the trauma survivor learns. There is nothing inherent in these models, however, that necessitates a *group* modality of treatment as opposed to an *individual* modality. Learning, whether of new patterns of thinking or new responses to previously feared stimuli, is the essential mechanism of change in cognitive and behavioral models.

Interpersonal and psychodynamic models of trauma focus on the relational and affective disturbances that arise from traumatic exposure. Interpersonally-oriented group treatment assists in the restoration of hope that connection with others is possible (Alexander, Neimeyere, Follette, Moore, & Harter, 1989). Cognitive and behavioral group treatments do not address directly the relational damage wrought by trauma. In interpersonal and dynamic group treatments, the process of sharing traumatic memories with other survivors instills commonality among individuals. Psychodynamically-inspired models encourage the exploration of affects and meanings associated with traumatic material (Roth, Dye, & Lebowitz, 1988). In both of these models, the process of sharing and altering

Table 1.1

Citation	Conceptual Model	Patient Population	Treatment Type	Methodology	Outcome Measures
Roth, Dye, & Lebowitz, 1988	Horowitz Stress Response	Adult sexual assault, incest survivors	High disclosure, trauma-focused group	Wait-list comparison	Modified Fear Survey (MFS); SCL-90; Social Adjustment Scale (SAS); Impact of Events Scale (IES)
Brom et al., 1989	Comparison among behavioral, dynamic, cognitive models	Women and men; wide range of trauma (sexual assault or incest identified)	Hypnosis, behavioral, or psychodynamic group tx.	Random assignment to dynamic, hypnosis, behavioral grp.; wait-list	SCL-90; State-Trait Anxiety; State-Trait Anger; Personality Questionnaire
Alexander et al., 1989	Interpersonal transaction	Women incest survivors (excluded those with suicidal ideation, psychosis)	Interpersonal transaction group (Yalom model)	Random assignment to wait-list control or to IT group	Beck Depression Inventory (BDI); SAS; SCL-90; MFS
Foa et al., 1995	Cognitive-behavioral model	Women survivors of sexual and non-sexual assault with PTSD	Brief Prevention Program; Assessment Control Grp.	No random assignment; participants in both grps. matched on PTSD severity; assault type; demographics	PTSD Scale (PSS); Standardized Assault Interview; BDI
Resick & Schnicke, 1992	Information-Processing Model	Women adult sexual assault survivors with PTSD sx (no competing pathology)	Cognitive Processing Therapy Group	No random assignment to wait-list; used a naturally occurring wait-list	SCL-90; IES; PSS; BDI, SAS, SCID-PTSD and SCID-Depression

3

affects and meaning within the context of a community (e.g., the group) is the mechanism of change.

While these models of trauma impact and intervention have advanced our understanding of the potential for change in trauma survivors, they are limited in a number of ways. First, they restrict clinicians' attention to relatively few areas of potential change. Cognitive-behavioral groups effectively reduce fear, anxiety, and depression (e.g., Brom, Skleber, & Defares, 1989; Chemtob, Novaco, Hamada, & Gross, 1997; Foa, Hearst-Ikeda, & Perry, 1995). The cognitive and behaviorally based studies outlined in Table 1.1 thus limit the target symptoms to fear, anxiety, and depression, symptoms of intrusion and avoidance. Group treatment outcome studies that examine interpersonal or psychodynamic models have included in their targets of change an individual's social or personality functioning in addition to fear, anxiety, and depression.

Another limitation in the models surveyed here is the implicit assumption that trauma survivors constitute a homogeneous group. Developmental and symptomatic heterogeneity suggests otherwise. Many groups exclude survivors, for instance, who are actively suicidal. These models offer little in the way of understanding the wide variation in the pretreatment clinical profiles of trauma survivors, or in the changes that individuals experience over time. Thus, the utility of group psychotherapy in the change process of whole, important areas of potential change in trauma survivors (e.g., dissociation, management of symptoms such as self-mutilation, memory) has been ignored in the empirical literature.

These models also offer little to elucidate the different responses that an individual might have to a particular intervention at a particular time. In the study of interpersonal treatment described by Alexander and her colleagues (1989), for instance, several participants dropped out of the study because they became suicidal and required hospitalization. An understanding of what treatment is useful for trauma survivors at what time is critical. Survivors who begin treatment with severe post-traumatic symptoms require treatment that focuses on the containment of intrusive memories and feelings. Later, as survivors have established a solid foundation of safety in their lives, they make better use of exploratory psychotherapy groups. Many of the treatment-outcome studies reviewed here draw upon a homogeneous group of trauma survivors. In these studies, samples consist largely of survivors of single-incident trauma, individuals without recent histories of inpatient psychiatric admissions, or individuals who are not actively self-harming. Yet some forms of group treatment may be quite helpful for this pool of trauma patients at early points in their recovery. Other forms of group treatment may be helpful at later points in their recovery. A comprehensive view of trauma and its wake should account for differences in traumatic presentation. Moreover, such a view of trauma should allow for an assessment of what type of treatment will be more helpful for what type of trauma survivor, at what point in time.

THERAPEUTIC RATIONALE

With concern for the variation in post-traumatic presentations and recognition of the need for different types of treatment at different times, clinical theorists at the Victims of Violence Program have developed a new model: The *Stages by Dimensions Model* of trauma recovery (Lebowitz, Harvey, & Herman, 1993). This model views recovery from trauma as a process that moves through three stages. In addition, recovery from trauma entails change along eight dimensions of psychological functioning. This model accounts for variation in functioning among acutely and chronically traumatized individuals. A stage-oriented model provides guidelines to clinicians with which to assess the right group for the right person at the right time.

In the first stage of recovery, the establishment of safety and self-care is the primary task. Safety begins with attention to the survivor's physical well-being. The survivor who is besieged by symptoms of hyperarousal or flashbacks, for instance, needs to cope with and reduce these symptoms so that she may feel her body is a safe place to inhabit. By assisting a survivor's ability to care for her body, the first stage restores a psychological sense of control. With this greater sense of control, the survivor's attention shifts to the creation of safety in her surrounding world. At this point, the clinician can encourage survivors to attend to the safety of their physical world (e.g., is their apartment secure or easy to break into) and to the safety of their relational world.

In the second stage, remembrance and mourning are central tasks. Traumatic memories may stand as the "black holes" described by survivors with full or partial amnesia, as visual images devoid of feeling, or as affective memories with no historical connections. The task of the second stage of recovery is to weave traumatic memory into the survivor's general life narrative in order to develop a more coherent sense of self. In the third stage, survivors attend to the repair of relationships with others in their immediate and wider community. The trauma story becomes one of several stories in a survivor's life. One's status as *survivor* no longer overshadows other aspects of one's identity.

At all stages of recovery, the psychological status of survivors may be assessed along the following eight domains of functioning:

1 *Authority over memory.* The process by which an individual experiences a sense of control over the remembering process. In this domain, survivors range from those who feel besieged by intrusive memories or have no access to memories, to those who feel that they can choose to remember events in their lives.

2 *Integration of memory with affect.* The extent to which a survivor experiences her memories as interwoven with feeling. Survivors may recall traumatic images without feeling or suffering from painful feelings uncontained by images. Others have memories that are braided with tolerable doses of negative affect and new affects that arise from contemporary understanding of the traumatic past.

3 *Affect tolerance.* The extent to which survivors can bear painful feelings. Survivors may present as unable to experience a range of feelings, as flooded by a few particular feelings, or as comfortable with positive as well as negative affect.

4 *Symptom mastery.* The degree to which survivors can anticipate, manage, contain, or prevent the cognitive and emotional disruption that arises from post-traumatic arousal.

5 *Self-esteem and self-care.* The degree to which survivors experience themselves as worthy of care and behave in ways that promote their best interest.

6 *Self-cohesion.* The extent to which survivors experience themselves as integrated or fragmented, in terms of thought, feeling, and action.

7 *Safe attachment.* The ability of the survivor to develop feelings of trust, safety, and enduring connection in relationships with others.

8 *Meaning-making.* The process of understanding what the survivor develops about himself or herself, in relation to the traumatic experience and to the world in which the trauma occurred.

Because the clinical presentations of all trauma survivors, regardless of their particular stage of recovery, can be conceptualized along these eight domains, the assessment of change is possible along a broad array of clinical issues. The *Stages by Dimensions Model* underlies group treatment at the Victims of Violence Program. This model also provides a concrete conceptual framework for the assessment of treatment efficacy.

PATIENT SELECTION

The notion of *Stages of Recovery* (Herman, 1992) helps significantly to predict which patients might respond positively to what type of group treatment. Individuals whose lives are characterized by instability, such as that arising from chronic suicidal ideation, impulses to harm themselves with self-mutilation or substance abuse, must attend to the creation of safety as their primary therapeutic task. Self-destructive (or other-destructive) action emerges when an individual is unable to contain powerful affects associated with trauma: anger, rage, and despair. Treatment for individuals with such presentations must assist in the development of cognitive, behavioral, and psychosocial skills that a survivor can use to contain and ultimately reduce the intensity of these overwhelming feelings. Survivors who are living in violent or dangerous situations, who are actively abusing substances, or who are actively psychotic, require the kind of clinical assistance that helps to strengthen their defenses and coping mechanisms. When these individuals are involved in groups that focus on the active disclosure of traumatic material, their own safety may be compromised. Moreover, the emotional safety of other group members, who have worked to create safety in their own lives, can be jeopardized by their anxiety about the person in the dangerous situation. These groups can be successful even when survivors vary in their trauma histories. Psychoeducation about post-traumatic stress disorder, for instance, can be useful whether the individual's symptoms arise from a single incident of assault in adulthood or chronic trauma in childhood.

Groups that focus on the active exploration of trauma histories are appropriate for individuals who have mastered the need to act on self-destructive impulses and who have been sober from substance abuse for a significant period of time. Trauma-focused groups are helpful for individuals who wish to work on integrating their feelings and memories about their past with their present lives. With the help of therapists, participants formulate a treatment goal that becomes the focus of their work in the group. Self-disclosure is high, and a strong sense of group cohesion develops as a result. These groups do not, however, rely heavily on the interpersonal process to promote positive change. Participants are encouraged to respond empathically to each other, and to assist each other in attaining their goals. Homogeneity in trauma-type and in patient gender is also helpful. Such a group, for instance, might consist of female rape survivors or male childhood sexual abuse survivors. Participants are not encouraged to work through interpersonal conflicts within the group.

Interpersonal process groups are helpful for individuals who are no longer overwhelmed by traumatic memories and affects. These groups can assist individuals who do not suffer significantly from intrusive or avoidant post-traumatic symptoms and who have a variety of feelings and a range of intensity in their feelings about their traumatic past. These groups allow for an examination of the more subtle effects of trauma on one's interpersonal functioning. Such groups need not consist solely of survivors of physical or sexual abuse, but they might include individuals who have had varied histories of emotional and interpersonal distress. These groups are most successful when participants have a relatively homogeneous range of functioning.

GROUP TREATMENT IN PRACTICE

Stage 1 Groups. At the Victims of Violence (VOV) Program, at The Cambridge Hospital, a group psychotherapy program based on the *Stages by Dimensions* model has been in effect for many years. Three groups are regarded as Stage 1 groups—groups that focus on the establishment of safety and self-care. All three groups have in common a didactic format, low interpersonal demand on the participants, and each requires little disclosure about details of one's trauma history. In fact, any significant degree of disclosure is actively discouraged.

The *Trauma Information* group is a psychoeducational group that essentially teaches individuals about post-traumatic sequelae. The goals of this group are to encourage an understanding of one's symptoms, to begin to foster toleration of feelings in the context of a group, and to develop a sense of safety with other people.

The *Safety and Self-Care* group is designed for individuals who actively harm themselves or otherwise care for themselves in inadequate or potentially destructive ways. The goals of this group are to develop skills of self-care, to manage and reduce impulses to harm oneself, and to improve one's sense of self-regard.

The *Stress Management* group is intended for individuals who would like to develop a sense of mastery over post-traumatic symptoms. Specific techniques for coping with symptoms such as flashbacks, dissociation, and depression are shared and discussed.

Stage 2 Groups.   The goals, structure, and clinical techniques of Stage 2 groups differ significantly from those of Stage 1 groups. First, the groups reflect the goals broadly mentioned previously, such as remembrance and mourning of the traumatic past. Survivors are asked to articulate a personal, specific goal prior to the onset of the group. In terms of the eight domains of functioning, improvement is expected in a survivor's ability to link affect with memory. With greater integration, a stronger sense of self-cohesion is expected. The retrieval of new memories is not a goal of these groups. Survivors sometimes find, however, that they can allow themselves to acknowledge previously ignored memories as they increase their capacity to tolerate painful feelings in the presence of other people. In this sense, then, survivors may develop a greater sense of authority over their memories. Stage 2 groups depend on a greater amount of self-disclosure about personal trauma histories than Stage 1 groups. Personal details are shared in a manner that is structured and goal-directed, rather than open-ended and exploratory (Herman, 1992). Currently, Stage 2 groups are structured to span 16, 24, or 36 weeks.

GUIDELINES FOR GROUP TREATMENT

To illustrate the process by which Stage 1 and Stage 2 groups at the Victims of Violence Program are formed, two types of groups will be discussed in depth.

Composite clinical vignettes will be provided to demonstrate the types of clinical choices and dilemmas encountered in this process.

Stage 1: Trauma Information Group.   This psychoeducational group was developed by Barbara Hamm, Psy.D. and Lois Glass, L.I.C.S.W. A treatment manual is underway (Glass, Hamm, & Koenan, in preparation). Group membership is open to men and women who have survived different types of trauma in childhood or adulthood. The group has been open to individuals who present with a range of psychological functioning. Recent psychiatric hospitalization is not an exclusionary criterion. Group members vary in their ability to give and take feedback in a group situation. This is an acceptable variation because the group process is not heavily dependent on such give and take. Group members should not be actively psychotic. Group members are required, however, to live in a safe situation and to be able to contract reliably against self-destructive behavior. Those members with histories of substance abuse must maintain sobriety. It is also recommended that individuals participate concurrently in individual psychotherapy. Prospective group members are screened in telephone interviews. The screening clinician (one of the two group leaders) requests permission to contact the individual therapist. The individual and group therapists should collaborate, together and with the client, to establish compatible treatment goals.

For many individuals, this group offers their first opportunity to sit in a room with other survivors. Shame is a cardinal affect among trauma survivors and is readily evoked by the company of others. The act of acknowledging to other people that one has been traumatized, therefore, takes tremendous courage. Initial entry into this group represents an opportunity to begin to master the experience of shame and a chance to break down its powerful hold on the survivor.

The Trauma Information Group runs for 10 weeks. Each session lasts an hour. The time-limited structure of the group adds to its ability to provide containment for individuals who are flooded with post-traumatic symptoms. In the group's first meeting, the structure, purpose, and rules of the group are explained. The importance of predictability is emphasized, and group members are asked to give notice well in advance if they must miss a group session. Group leaders and members introduce themselves briefly. At each subsequent session, the group begins with a check-in, as each member notes his or her reactions to the material discussed the previous week. In the initial round of introductions, group members are asked not to provide many details about their traumatic experiences. This request is explained to individuals during the screening process as well. Members are reminded that the goals of the group are to learn about post-traumatic sequelae and the process of recovery from trauma.

Each week, the group leaders lead a discussion about a particular topic after the initial check-in. Such topics include (a) understanding post-traumatic stress symptoms; (b) recognizing and coping with anger; and (c) understanding trust and the ways in which trauma impairs one's ability to trust. Group leaders distribute information sheets and worksheets about the topic of the day. Worksheets provide survivors with structured tasks that help them apply the didactic material to their own lives (Glass, Hamm, & Koenan, in preparation).

This didactic format provides survivors with a cognitive understanding of trauma and its sequelae. This understanding assuages survivors' fears that their symptoms are evidence that they are "crazy." Post-traumatic symptoms thus become recognizable, but also ego-alien—in other words, understood as connected to the violence that was inflicted upon them rather than connected to their own flaws. Feelings of alienation and isolation erode when survivors recognize that their responses to trauma are common, human responses to atrocious circumstances.

After group leaders present the topic of the day, an open discussion of the issues is held among the group. The primary clinical challenge for group leaders in this portion of a session is to encourage group members to apply the material to their own lives, to allow for discussion of that application, and simultaneously to assist members in keeping contained in-depth discussion of traumatic material. When this dilemma emerges, group leaders need to redirect the discussion carefully and respectfully, so that group members do not feel that they are being silenced once again. Reminders about the process of recovery, the need for self-protection and pacing, can assist toward these ends.

Ideally, participants leave this group with a greater understanding of the effects of trauma on their lives. This understanding places their symptomatology within the context of a post-traumatic reaction. With this knowledge, strategies for managing painful affects or intrusive symptoms can be developed. Material that may have once seemed abstract has been digested and applied to their lives. Sometimes, participants benefit from attending the group for a second time. This has been especially helpful for those survivors who felt particularly uncomfortable, initially, sitting with other survivors. For these survivors, although their discomfort may have lessened over the course of 10 weeks, their ability to attend to the material was compromised. Thus, they gained some mastery over the experience of shame, but they wished for another chance to relearn the didactic material.

Stage 2: Trauma-Focused Groups. Trauma-focused groups were developed for survivors who have created safety in their lives and who are ready to explore traumatic memories in some depth (Herman, 1992). These groups require a more intensive screening process than Stage 1 groups. Prospective group members are interviewed in person by the two group leaders. In these interviews, clinicians assess carefully a survivor's ability to maintain safety. Contact with prospective group members' individual therapists is essential in conducting a responsible evaluation. Prospective group members should have had some previous experience in a group treatment situation, preferably on an outpatient basis.

In the initial interview, prospective group members are asked to articulate a treatment goal. Members may receive feedback from the group leaders and their individual therapists about the formulation of their treatment goal. Because this group depends on personal disclosure and exploration of one's trauma history, members may be at risk of discussing traumatic material in a way that creates greater anxiety and may precipitate flashbacks. By creating a clearly articulated treatment goal, members can focus their discussion of personal material in a way that is explicitly linked to a desired outcome. Because the group is time-limited, the creation of goals allows group members to direct their work in the group toward particular ends. At the point of termination, group members can evaluate their own progress toward this particular goal.

The goals that prospective group members bring to their initial interview are often somewhat vague. One individual might wish to "work on" her anger; another might wish to "work on having feelings" when she thinks about her traumatic experiences. In the initial interview and in early group sessions, leaders and members assist the individual in making the goal more concrete. Working on her anger might take the form of reviewing one traumatic incident in detail in the group, describing her emotional reactions at the time, and findings ways to connect the affect of anger to her experience. Likewise, the individual who wishes to "work on having feelings" might share one traumatic incident with the group and use the group's input to understand the wide variety of feelings she might have had at the time.

The structure of a Stage 2 group differs from that of a Stage 1 group in several ways. In a Stage 2 group, the emphasis is on the participation of group members and their opportunity to talk with each other about their experiences. Group leaders structure the group by describing ground rules in the initial session, citing the need for predictability in attendance, requesting advance notice if any group members plans to miss a group, emphasizing the need for confidentiality, and so on. Group leaders inform members about the structure of the group during the interview process but review the format in the initial group session. Group members are informed, for instance, that the group begins with a check-in, a process by means of which all group members share their current affect states, as well as their wishes to take time in the group that week. In the first two or three weeks, group members take time to share information about their trauma history. In a sense, all members tell their trauma story to the group. In the following weeks, the remainder of the session following the initial check-in is divided among two or three group members who wish to work on their goal. In the last two weeks, group members take time to share thoughts and feelings about termination.

> Mary is a 29-year-old woman who has been in individual therapy for two years. As a child between the ages of 6 and 10, she was sexually abused by a brother. She first sought the assistance of a psychotherapist when she began having flashbacks of this abuse. Mary knew nothing of flashbacks and felt she was "going crazy." Mary was terrified of sharing any of her history with anyone; she often told her therapist that she was to blame for her abuse because her perpetrator was only several years older than she was. With her therapist's support, she enrolled in a psychoeducational group about trauma. In this setting, Mary did not need to tackle her feelings of shame and self-blame directly with others. Instead, she was allowed to listen and learn about the symptoms of post-traumatic stress disorder. She was able to identify her experiences as a coherent syndrome that is common among individuals who have been victimized.
>
> Two years later, Mary had made considerable progress in her treatment. She no longer felt overwhelmed by anxiety attacks or flashbacks on a regular basis. She knew what situations made her anxious or triggered flashbacks, and she was able to prepare herself for these experiences. She felt more able to manage greater responsibility at work and was starting to feel better about herself than she had in a long time.
>
> Although Mary's "symptoms" had been considerably reduced, she continued to hold a core set of beliefs about her abuse that allowed for the persistence of intense shame. These feelings seemed to create a stumbling block for her in work and relationships. Despite some of the more positive ways in which she felt about herself, she confided in her therapist that she felt that most people would revile her if they truly knew her. Although her therapist knew most of the details of her trauma history, this sharing did not significantly alter Mary's sense of shame. She argued that her therapist had to accept her because that was her job.
>
> At this stage in Mary's recovery, a trauma-focused group was indicated. Her therapist believed that Mary would benefit from the support and acceptance of peers, who might challenge Mary's self-negating thoughts and feelings. Mary's initial goal in the group was to "learn to feel better about herself." Over time, Mary was able to identify specific thoughts and feelings about herself that arose from particular characteristics of her trauma history. She was able to talk about, for example, the fact that she sometimes experienced physical pleasure when her brother molested her. Other group members identified with the confusing, painful experiences of unwanted, coerced

sexual response. For Mary, the knowledge that other women had similar responses at times to situations similar to hers went a long way in helping her to shift her beliefs and feelings about her role in her abuse.

CONCLUSION

The merits of a multidimensional, stage-oriented approach to the understanding of trauma impact and its treatment are multiple. This model recognizes the variation in clinical profiles evident among trauma survivors. It provides, however, a systematic method by which to organize clinical decision-making for this heterogeneous population. The *Stages by Dimensions* model of group treatment provides a method by means of which to focus treatment on particular aspects of the process of recovery from trauma while recognizing that the needs for clinical assistance of each trauma survivor changes over time.

Mary could not have benefited from this trauma-focused group unless she already possessed considerable skill in managing symptoms such as affect-flooding. This vignette illustrates the need for careful attention to timing in the treatment of trauma survivors. Moreover, a *Stages by Dimensions* model of trauma recovery allows clinicians not only to attend to appropriate timing but also to hone in on particular aspects of post-traumatic sequelae. This model allows for the articulation of specific treatment goals, enabling survivors like Mary to aim for particular outcomes in their therapeutic work. Clinicians can use this model for treatment planning, and as a conceptual framework by which to evaluate a person's progress in treatment.

The *Stages by Dimensions* model of trauma recovery is particularly useful for clinicians who work with individuals who have experienced multiple forms of trauma at different points in their lives. The model assists clinicians in tailoring treatment plans that are sensitive to a client's place in his or her recovery process. The model also provides an organizational structure for group treatment that is sensitive in this same way. Future treatment outcome studies are needed to examine the effects of group treatment that are organized around the stages of trauma recovery and around a variety of psychological dimensions relevant to trauma recovery. We need to examine the effects of group treatment on outcome variables of broader significance than symptom reduction. Studies that include outcome measures on affect management, self-representations, and interpersonal attachments are some of the outcome criteria highlighted by this model. The effects of different types of group structure and process on clinical outcomes would also be a welcome addition to the group psychotherapy literature. The *Stages by Dimensions* framework offers one such conceptual scheme with which to examine these questions.

REFERENCES

Alexander, P., Neimeyer, R. A., Follette, V. M., Moore, M. K., & Harter, S. (1989). A comparison of group treatments of women sexually abused as children. *Journal of Consulting and Clinical Psychology, 57,* 479–483.

Brom, D., Kleber, R. J., & Defares, P. B. (1989). Brief psychotherapy for post-traumatic stress disorders. *Journal of Consulting and Clinical Psychology, 57,* 607–612.

Chemtob, C. M., Novaco, R. W., Hamada, R. S., & Gross, D. M. (1997). Cognitive-behavioral treatment for severe anger in post-traumatic stress disorder. *Journal of Consulting and Clinical Psychology, 65,* 184–189.

Foa, E. B., Hearst-Ikeda, D., & Perry, K. J. (1995). Evaluation of a brief cognitive-behavioral program for the prevention of PTSD in recent assault victims. *Journal of Clinical and Consulting Psychology, 63,* 948–955.

Glass, L., Hamm, B., & Koenen, K. (in preparation). *A treatment manual for a trauma information group.* Unpublished manuscript.

Harvey, M. R. (1996). An ecological view of psychological trauma and trauma recovery. *Journal of Traumatic Stress, 9,* 3–23.

Herman, J. L. (1992). *Trauma and recovery.* New York: Basic Books.

Koss, M. P., & Harvey, M. R. (1991). *The rape victim: Clinical and community interventions.* Newbury Park, CA: Sage.

Lebowitz, L., Harvey, M. R., & Herman, J. L. (1993). A stage-by-dimension model of recovery from sexual trauma. *Journal of Interpersonal Violence, 8,* 378–391.

Resick, P. A., & Schnicke, M. K. (1992). Cognitive processing therapy for sexual assault victims. *Journal of Consulting and Clinical Psychology, 60,* 748–756.

Roth, S., Dye, E., & Lebowitz, L. (1988). Group therapy for sexual assault victims. *Psychotherapy, 25,* 82-93.

Schatzow, E., & Herman, J. L. (1989). Breaking secrecy: Adult survivors disclose to their families. *Psychiatric Clinics of North America, 12,* 337–349.

Chapter 2

Family as a Group Treatment for PTSD

Don R. Catherall

It may seem odd at first to include the family in a book on group treatment of PTSD. But, perhaps, it will seem odd for only a moment. For, when you stop and think about it, the family is the first and foremost group in our society. Most of the conceptualizations about groups are either drawn from the family, expressed in the form of metaphors of the family, or readily transferable to the family. Family systems theory is basically a group theory. Its explanations about the behavior of individuals emphasize their mutual influence upon one another, as opposed to an emphasis on sources within individuals.

GROUP PREMISES OF A FAMILY APPROACH

There are a number of premises that have developed in the area of family therapy which bear on group processes. These premises have historically established family therapy's focus on the interpersonal dimension and the influence family members exert upon one another.

The Family Group Is the Patient

The first premise of a family orientation is that what affects one member of the group affects all members of the group. One of the early steps in the establishment of a family approach was Nathan Ackerman's (1937) observation that the family is a unit and can be viewed as a whole unto itself. Individuals' behavior can be understood as a function of both their individual experience and their participation as a member of the family group (Loukas, Twitchell, Piejak, Fitzgerald, & Zucker, 1998). This view of the family as a group has implications for both the effects of traumatic stress and recovery from traumatic stress. When an individual is traumatized, the entire family is affected. Recovery is both an individual and a family process, not simply the task of the affected member.

Group Behavior Is Rule-Governed

Another premise of a family orientation is that the members of the family system are operating according to rules that govern the entire system (Jackson, 1957, 1965). Thus, the rules are not set by one individual and are not wholly under the control of one individual. Rather, everyone is operating within a system of rules that exceeds the grasp of any single member. Change can thus be sought by addressing the rules themselves, rather than trying to change individuals. Therapists can produce profound effects by focusing on the rules of the system or group. This way of thinking has influenced numerous other group approaches, almost all of which make a point of clarifying and identifying the operant rules of the group.

Individual Experience Is a Function of the Group Relational Structure

Still another premise of a family orientation is that there is an underlying structure to the family group and the effect of changing the structure is similar to the effect of changing the rules. The structure is inherent in the relationships among the members of the group (Hinde, 1995), and it is supported by the operant rules. Again, family therapists believe that altering the underlying structure of a relationship, such as a dominant-submissive relationship, will alter the behavior and experience of the individuals in the relationship (Minuchin, 1974).

Structure Can Be Observed in Recurring Patterns of Communication

Another premise of the family approach is that the structure of relationships underlying a longstanding intact group is inherent in observable patterns of communication among the group members (Watzlawick, Beavin, & Jackson, 1967). Thus, family therapists watch to see who says what to whom. The point of looking at communication in this way is to see beyond the content of the communication and glean what the communication says about the relationship between the communicators (Haley, 1963). More than 30 years ago, Singer and Wynne (1965) were able to predict the diagnoses of schizophrenic young adults through analyzing the communication transactions of their parents.

GROUP PROCESSES OBSERVED IN THE FAMILY

There are a number of phenomena that have been observed in families that have informed therapists' thinking about people's behavior.

Triangles

The understanding of dyadic behavior is often enhanced by taking a triadic point of view. Family therapists were among the first to recognize that the meaning of a transaction between two individuals may change if one studies the effect upon a third individual who is involved with the two individuals (Minuchin, 1974). A third person is often brought into a dyadic relationship in a family as a means of modifying the dyadic relationship (Wagner & Reiss, 1995). For example, a mother might initiate conflict with the son in order to engage a distant father.

Roles

Another group phenomenon that was originally observed in families is how individuals acquire roles (Ackerman, 1954). The idea of a role bridges the gap between individual personality and the influence of the social environment (Ackerman & Behrens, 1956). Roles facilitate the accomplishment of group tasks; they provide structure for the group and sources of identity for individual group members. In families, individuals often accept negative roles (e.g., scapegoat, acting out child) in order to preserve the functioning of the overall family group.

Attitudes and Beliefs

Another group phenomenon that is perhaps seen most clearly in families is the consensual reality that is maintained within the family group. A belief system of attitudes and attributions develops that contributes to the ways in which family members perceive and experience their interactions with others, including people outside the family. Minuchin (1979) targeted this family belief system as a central focus of therapeutic intervention.

Emotional Support

For this discussion of the family and PTSD, perhaps the most important of the many group processes that are captured best in the family is the group's role in providing emotional support to affected members. Nowhere is this support more important than in one's own family. Research on emotional support has highlighted its central importance in coping with and recovering from exposure to trauma (McCubbin & Figley, 1983).

Dealing with Emotion as a Group

As important as the family's provision of emotional support to individual members are the complicated processes through which members of a family group cooperate and collude in the processing of emotions (Gottman, Katz, & Hooven, 1996; Yalom, 1985). It was in families that therapists first demonstrated how members could unconsciously work together to create and maintain an emotional state, such as anger, in order to collectively avoid an emotional state perceived as more disabling, such as grief (Paul & Grosser, 1965). The parents play the pivotal role in this process, influencing the children's ability to recognize, express and regulate most emotions (Free, Alechina, & Zahn-Waxler, 1996).

WORKING WITH THE FAMILY STRUCTURE

The relational structure of the family, as expressed in their interactions in the therapist's presence, is the central focus of the therapy. The therapist observes that structure in order to identify maladaptive patterns, such as the existence of family secrets (Stiver, 1990b). As the maladaptive patterns are identified, the therapist educates the family and suggests changes. When the family is unable to implement changes, the therapist intensifies the focus and explores the roots of the difficulty. If the difficulty involves interpersonal issues, the therapist attempts to facilitate corrective interaction. For example, "Tell your husband how you feel about what he did." If the difficulty involves intrapersonal issues, the therapist works through the traditional tools of empathy, interpretation, confrontation, clarification, and support.

In the case of families with traumatized members, the maladaptive patterns sought are those that interfere with an effective recovery environment. Thus, a variety of relational structures might become the focus of the therapist's efforts. These can include situations like: rigid roles (that prevent members from responding adequately); dysfunctional rules (that disallow revealing vulnerability or grieving); difficulties managing strong emotions (that interfere with telling trauma stories); triangles (that prevent resolution of interpersonal problems); inappropriate power structures (that disempower and obstruct problem-solving); and irrational beliefs (that keep individuals from feeling safe).

THE ROLE OF THE THERAPIST

The role of the therapist working with a family contains the same fundamentals as that of the group therapist. In both situations, the therapist is concerned with the members' ability to function as a cohesive whole, i.e., as a group. The therapist works to help members overcome difficulties—usually relational or interactive in nature—that interfere with effective, cohesive group functioning. The therapist does this primarily by facilitating interactions between group or family members. At times, the therapist takes an educational role and defines norms and a point of view about the group or family. In these ways, group and family therapists have a similar role, sort of a cross between a traffic cop and a teacher.

However, there are important differences between the usual group and a family. The family therapist is dealing with a group that has the specific task of nurturing and maintaining its members. It is different from other groups in that it is an intact group, with a lifetime membership for each member and a history that goes back generations (Scabini & Cigoli, 1998). It is a group held together by the strongest of bonds. It is a group with a highly structured definition, marked by kinship patterns, cultural norms, gender roles, etc. It has the most vulnerable, undifferentiated members of any group (young children), and some members can have tremendous power over other members.

The family therapist is not creating a group and declaring the norms; he or she is joining a group and learning their norms. The family therapist can only be effective by recognizing the existing structure of the family and working within it. In order to have any real influence, the therapist must be allowed to become a part of the family, at least temporarily. Minuchin (1974) refers to this as "joining" the family.

THE IMPACT OF TRAUMA ON THE FAMILY

All the above dimensions of family life, and more, are relevant when an individual in the family has been traumatized. The family approach leads us to expect that the traumatization of one family member means that the entire family will have been affected. This effect usually reverberates throughout the relationships in the family. Since recovery from traumatization generally requires a high level of expressivity and cohesion in the traumatized individual's supportive relationships, the family can usually be expected to have difficulty if they are operating according to constrictive rules in these areas. Family therapists observe the patterns of communication—in addition to hearing the family's self-report—in order to determine whether there are obstructive elements in the structure of the family.

New Stress on Old Wounds

The traumatization of a family member not only poses new problems for a family, it often stirs up many of the family's old conflicts. The clear need for emotional support of the traumatized member can surface longstanding difficulties in the family's capacity to attend to the needs of individual members. Feelings of jealousy, resentment, and anger often accompany a call to crisis in the service of a single member.

In order to cope with the impact of the trauma—both the impact upon the affected member and the impact upon the entire family group—the family must function together as a team. The ability to function as a team is often impeded by old roles and patterns of functioning that emphasize relational positioning over other needs of members.

Problems Managing Emotion

Perhaps most telling in a family that has been adversely affected by trauma (a traumatized family) is the great difficulty they have managing certain emotions. Feelings of helplessness, hopelessness, sadness, and rage are difficult to manage—whether by an individual or an entire family. The family can work together to express and share such feelings or the members can unconsciously collude in avoiding the recognition and expression of such distressing feelings (Danieli, 1985). Ineffective coping leads to increased avoidance of such feelings through conflict and distance.

Conflict and Blame

The family copes best when they face difficult feelings and situations without blaming individuals. When the family is colluding in avoidance, they generally fall into some form of denial or acting out. Often, conflict in the family serves to detour the group away from unacceptable emotional states that are associated with the traumatization. These conflicts usually center on an individual or relationship in the family. Thus, interrupting blame patterns and facilitating genuine affective communication form the substance of many therapy sessions.

Management of Shame

Strong feelings of shame are often mobilized by trauma. When members are resistant to recognizing and acknowledging their feelings of shame, they often resort to strategies that create conflict within the family. Nathanson (1992) asserts that individuals have predictable response styles to shame: (a) withdrawal, (b) attacking self, (c) avoidance, and (d) attacking others. Each of these places a different kind of stress on the family. The alternative is open, accepting communication. When this kind of communication is not achieved, then shame is avoided through these mechanisms and relational issues predominate.

The Camouflage of Secondary Problems

The family distress spawned by traumatic stress generally leads to secondary problems, such as conflict, triangulation, and distancing. The therapist who is not aware of the nature of the original blow to the family—the traumatization of one or more members—may mistakenly view these secondary issues as the primary problem. Indeed, it is important to attend to these real problems but it is also important to get beyond them to the trauma-related issues. This is the area in which the family first got off track in their recovery. Instead of coping effectively, they resorted to some form of dysfunctional coping—such as substance abuse—and both failed to resolve the trauma and created new problems in the process.

Secondary Traumatization of Other Family Members

Everyone in the family is vulnerable to developing secondary traumatization (Figley, 1995). As in any group situation in which the distressing experience of some member(s) is deemed threatening, some family members are likely to protect themselves by distancing from the affected member. They achieve distance by focusing on their differences from the affected member, thereby not truly relating to the affected member's experience. This makes it easier for them to believe that they would not respond similarly if they had been in the survivor's situation (Catherall, 1991).

This focus on difference is sometimes characterized as a stage in group development, but it is helpful to think of it as a defensive strategy in groups. It can develop any time a group must deal with the contagious potential of a member's emotional state (Jaques, 1955).

Adding to the Relational Trauma

When family members focus on differences from the affected member(s), it increases the affected member's feelings of alienation. The social distancing of potential supporters constitutes an additional trauma for the survivor, a relational trauma (Catherall, 1989; Symonds, 1980). The result is that the survivor ends up feeling that there is something wrong with him rather than that something terrible has happened to him. Subjectively, this contributes to the survivor's experience of shame.

The Danger of Staying Connected

On the other hand, family members who do not distance from the affected member are at risk for being affected themselves. In effect, every family member's personal schemas of the world can be altered by the influence of the affected member (McCann and Pearlman, 1990). As more and more members are affected, the cognitive map of the world maintained by the family as a whole will change as well. Children brought up in that environment will learn that new map, and so the cycle of a traumatized family will be set in place through the generations.

The issue of distancing from versus relating to the survivor's experience occurs in every group involving survivors (Catherall, 1995). The other group members are always motivated to protect themselves from secondary traumatization. But they are also motivated to relate to and help support the survivor. This is particularly true when the group is held together by the intimate bonds of family relationships. Thus, there is usually conflict over how much to relate to the affected member(s). The conflict is often externalized and acted out between family members.

THE RECOVERY PROCESS

The family can be the optimal healing sanctuary for a trauma survivor. If a survivor is with loved ones who are understanding, tolerant, supportive, attuned to the survivor's emotional needs, and able to bear their own troubled feelings, then there can be no better healing environment. A natural process of recovery from traumatization occurs as the survivor examines his or her experience in the safety of the trust relationships with the other family members (Catherall, 1992; Herman, 1992).

The family often helps the survivor by serving as part of a protective barrier referred to as the *trauma membrane*, a term first coined by Lindy (1985) to describe the survivor's activities to fend off people who are "unfamiliar with the particular absurd meaning of the trauma and who might serve to stimulate unwanted traumatic memories without a constructive context for healing" (Lindy, 1986, p. 200). As with a cast on a broken limb, the trauma membrane can become an impediment to healing if it remains in place too long.

Recovery conditions are optimal when trauma survivors have an interpersonal environment in which they can safely discuss and examine their reactions to their traumatic experience. The process of recovery is an emotional process. When family members are able to connect with survivors with regard to their powerful feelings, then the survivor is held and the family gets closer. The primary job of the therapist is to facilitate the establishment and maintenance of a safe recovery environment.

The underlying principle is that the family provides the healing experience. Thus, the therapist's job is the same as in so many other forms of group therapy. It is to facilitate the group process, relying upon the group itself to provide the healing experience.

The affected individual comes to feel more normal as he or she is held (emotionally) by the family group. This interrupts the onset of feelings of alienation and lowered self esteem. As affected members feel stronger and supported by the family groups, they are more able to find the discipline and courage to make needed lifestyle changes, to examine the terrible thoughts and feelings associated with the trauma, and to accept a more benign and realistic perspective on themselves and their experience (Figley, 1989). But this normal healing process occurs only when the family is able to employ effective coping strategies in dealing with stressors.

Effective Versus Ineffective Coping

McCubbin and Figley (1983) examined families and differentiated those that coped effectively from those that did not. They note that families both react to and produce stress, thus either undermining (via ineffective coping) or contributing to (via effective coping) the functioning of individual members. Effective coping in a family means that the family group approaches the trauma of individual members as a problem for the entire family, not as an indication of something inherently defective about the affected individual. The family basically communicates the message that there is not something wrong with the affected member, his experience is a normal response to an abnormal situation (Frank, 1961; Ochberg, 1991).

Ineffective coping is seen in the following areas (McCubbin and Figley, 1983):

Ineffective problem solving. The family is unable to identify stressors effectively, and does not utilize resources well.

Lack of physical safety. The family does not provide an atmosphere of safety for the more vulnerable members. This is seen in the prevalence of violence or substance abuse or both.

Lack of emotional safety. The family does not provide an atmosphere of emotional safety. As a group, the family tends to approach problems by assigning blame rather than seeking solutions. Problems are seen as centered in individuals rather than accepted as problems for the entire family. Unspoken shame shapes many of the interactions that occur in the family.

Communication problems. Communication is not open. It is usually indirect, and there is little tolerance for idiosyncratic expressions and behavior.

Problems in the family structure. The entire family group lacks cohesion. Individuals are cast in rigid roles. The boundaries between subsystems are either diffuse or overly rigid.

When the family falls into any or all of the above coping patterns, its members lose their ability to operate as a cohesive group and provide a healing environment for the affected individual or the secondarily affected members or both. Once the family starts failing to cope well, many dimensions of family life are disrupted.

The overall atmosphere of the family becomes sterile and unauthentic, lacking the closeness and connection that characterizes groups of people who are intimately involved with one another.

A TRAUMATIZED FAMILY

In traumatized families, the breakdown of a supportive, cohesive group combines with the impediments to open communication and other ineffective coping strategies to cause the development of secondary problems and disruption of the family's normal healing capacity. These are the areas of focus for family therapy. The goal of the family therapist is to remove or resolve these obstacles so that normal processes of healing can move forward.

ORIENTATION AND GOALS OF FAMILY THERAPY

The family therapist's patient is the entire family group. The therapist is concerned with the ability of the family members to operate as a cohesive unit. The family therapist's interventions are thus directed at group phenomena such as interactions among members, shared perceptions and beliefs of members (or conflict between perceptions and beliefs of members), and group tasks.

The primary group task required of every family is the caretaking of family members. Cusinato (1998) identifies three key variables that define parental caretaking style: warmth, control, and consistency. All of these are subject to change in the wake of trauma. If parents are personally numb, then they become less warm. If they feel out of control, they often become more controlling of the children (and even of each other). And any of these kinds of changes constitute changes in consistency.

If the parents are in conflict and a child has stepped into the role of caretaker, then several family group processes may need correcting. The child may have been triangulated into the inappropriate role in order to stabilize the parents' conflict. Thus, the parents may need to resolve their conflict in order to become emotionally accessible and relieve the child of the inappropriate role. This constitutes a structural change. It would likely include changing the rules that developed to support the altered structure, rules which affect everyone in the family.

The therapist arrives at the therapeutic focus by working backward from the desired state of functioning, i.e., asking what prevents the family from effectively taking care of its members. This then leads to the roles, rules, triangulation, and parental conflict. In effect, the parental conflict is not seen as the problem; the family's failure to provide appropriate caretaking is the problem. The parental conflict is simply one of the factors contributing to the family's failure to provide caretaking. The conflict itself may not have to be resolved, but the family must find a way of coping with it that does not disrupt the group task of caretaking.

Some of the central areas in traumatized families that have been identified as being amenable to group or family level intervention are: (a) the family's disrupted capacity to take care of its members, (b) the set of trauma-influenced beliefs, attitudes, and attributions that comprise the family perception, (c) the family's lost experience of safety, (d) the interpersonal effects of symptomatic members, (e) the continued effects of the trauma itself, and (f) the affected elements of the family structure (Catherall, 1998). In addition to these is the acquisition of more effective coping strategies; therapists generally educate families about better strategies for coping.

The family can be regarded as functional when the impoverished atmosphere changes and the members once more operate as a supportive, cohesive group.

The Family's Disrupted Capacity to Take Care of Its Members

One of the primary functions of every family group is to take care of the physical and emotional needs of individual members, particularly children. In the wake of traumatization, there is a breakdown in the family's capacity to identify, express, and contain powerful feelings. Krystal (1988) has discussed the development of alexithymia among individuals; at the family level, this contributes to a lack of emotional attunement and responsiveness between family members.

In families with children, the worst disruptions are seen in the emotional inaccessibility of the parents and the parentification of the children (Stiver, 1990a). The parents are unable to provide the full spectrum of parenting, usually leaving significant gaps in nurturance, modeling, limit-setting, managing resources, and perhaps most commonly, being emotionally accessible. Some children try to fulfill these gaps by becoming some variant of a parentified child (e.g., an emotional caretaker, surrogate spouse, breadwinner, homemaker), while others adopt irresponsible roles that express the family's conflicts and draw attention to the denied feelings and needs.

The goal of the therapy is to help the family resume taking care of the needs of the members. This includes attending to the family's ability to deal with the distressing emotions related to the traumatization. Since the appropriate structure is for the adults to take care of the children (and sometimes older generations), the therapy may have to pursue structural changes and shift people in or out of roles. Mainly, the goal is to remove the impediments to the family's performance of the caretaking task.

The Family Reality

Every group develops its own unique view of reality by shaping and mutually reinforcing each other's views through such processes as agreement, challenge, skepticism, reward, and punishment. The result of these processes is a convergence in the group's consensual view of reality or family perception (Figley, 1998). The more closed the family is, the less heterogeneous the consensual reality, and the more likely it will diverge from the reality orientation of the surrounding culture. The social avoidance and alienation dimensions of individual traumatization tend to interfere with the family's ability to maintain an open system. Thus, many traumatized families are closed off and maintain an internal reality that is at odds with that of the surrounding culture.

The internal reality of the traumatized family is strongly influenced by family stories and myths related to the trauma and often contains a worldview that makes it difficult for members to play a productive role in society. By addressing issues such as who we are, how we behave, what we believe, and what the themes are that define our lives, family stories play a role in the self-definition of family members. New members and acquaintances of the family are usually introduced to the family's self-definition through the medium of the family stories.

Family myths are the lessons that are gleaned from the traumatic events in the family stories. The family myth usually entails decisions that had short term value, such as to do or say nothing that might upset the survivor, but which can interfere with normal family life when continued indefinitely (Kramer, 1985). The family myth is often at the center of those trauma membrane activities which carry on for too long.

When the worldview of a family has been adversely affected by traumatization, it is usually reflected in rigid and excessive safety concerns, difficulty trusting others, negative self-concepts, and poor self-esteem among family members. The therapist's role is to help the family see how these beliefs and attitudes developed as a result of the trauma and to provide the safety of the therapeutic setting so that the family can explore alternative operational hypotheses about their world. If the family is excessively closed, the therapist may attempt to influence the family to become more open to the outside culture.

Safety Concerns

Every group must concern itself with safety. An intense, intimate group like the family is concerned about the safety of its members both inside and outside the group. But every group must deal with the issue of safety within the group. The primary source of danger inside the group is the possibility of damage to the self. The family can support and enrich each member, or it can drain and erode the self-definition of members. It is not very likely that a family will be able to support some members while inflicting damage on others. When a family develops an atmosphere of blaming and criticism, even the members inflicting the negative input are not free to grow.

Traumatized families may sustain considerable concern about the physical safety of members. People who have been traumatized continue to feel vulnerable to similar future trauma, even after the primary symptoms of PTSD have remitted (Greening & Dollinger, 1992). They often develop attitudes of distrust, cynicism, and suspiciousness, as well as reliance upon defenses like denial. But it is the fear of fully revealing oneself within the family that leaves the most constricting grip on the growth of family members. In an unsafe environment, it is not safe to expose parts of the self that will be held as shameful by other group members.

Hence, a central aspect of the family therapy is to establish a nonblaming, nonjudgmental atmosphere that can make it possible for members to share those vulnerable parts of themselves. The family therapist must actively block any shaming or blaming behaviors, while doing so in such a way as to not cause the individual whose behavior is being interrupted to feel shamed or blamed.

The Effects of Symptomatic Members

The presence of members with Post-Traumatic Stress Disorder (PTSD) symptoms places stress on the other family members. Arousal-related symptoms—including sleep problems, irritability, rage attacks, workaholism (and alcoholism, which is often associated with the direct arousal symptoms)—place immediate demands on the other family members. Avoidance symptoms, particularly social avoidance, have a major impact on the family's freedom and daily life. Loved ones often end up in the bind of feeling resentful if they withdraw along with the afflicted member(s) but guilty if they continue with their lives and leave the afflicted member(s) behind. The reexperiencing symptoms are frightening and frequently develop in such a way that other family members are drawn into playing regular roles in reenactments associated with the trauma.

The family therapist normalizes the stressful experience of the other family members. The family may need assistance (a) developing strategies for dealing with the affected members's arousal symptoms, (b) establishing a workable struc-ture so that other members can go on with their lives without abandoning the affected member, and (c) disentangling members from the survivor's reenactments.

Continued Traumatic Effects

The family that is dominated by traumatic themes is like a phonograph record that gets stuck and keeps repeating the same sound. The family seems to be stuck in the loop of failing to process the traumatic event effectively. Instead, the traumatic event remains in the center of family life, veiled in the repetitious references to it. Various members of the family get caught in roles associated with the event and play their parts endlessly as well. The therapist must interrupt the roles if the family group is to be able to bring a different ending to the repetitions.

But, whereas the traumatic event seems to repeat endlessly in some families, it dominates by its absence in others. Many people who grow up in traumatized families live lives defined by the trauma, though it is never openly discussed or acknowledged. Herman has noted how the recovery of individual survivors often includes a survivor mission related to the trauma (1992). This mission becomes an organizing principle for their lives. In families affected by trauma, overcoming the effects of the traumatization can become the principle that organizes the lives of everyone in the family. Family members may acquire missions for a variety of reasons. Those reasons may include giving meaning to the trauma, making up for it, proving the family's worth, or perhaps ensuring that the trauma can never be repeated. In a family that does not openly discuss or acknowledge the effects of the trauma, members acquire missions which they do not understand even while they feel compelled to pursue them.

Family therapy can create the opportunity for a dialogue among family members, a chance to discuss issues that may not have been approachable before. The therapist can direct the discussion toward a deeper understanding of the family's self-definition, including the roots of many of the family's core values and beliefs. This process facilitates the exploration of issues such as the extent to which family members grow up with a sense of mission related to their family.

CASE EXAMPLE

The G. Family consisted of four members, Mr. and Mrs. G. and their two sons. The first son was four years older than the second son, who was born with birth defects. The birth defects were serious, but Mr. and Mrs. G. were told that they could be remediated by surgery when the boy was older. They were led to believe the surgery would be relatively straightforward. When the boy was four years old, the surgery was conducted. Unexpected complications arose. The boy nearly died as a result of the first surgery and ended up requiring a series of operations. He was in a precarious state for approximately one year, and required special care at home for another year. He eventually survived the surgeries, though with some permanent disabilities, particularly deafness.

Mr. and Mrs. G. sought therapy during the second year of the intensive home care. At that point, the older boy was nine and the younger boy was five years old. The presenting problems were marital conflict and an emotional involvement between Mrs. G. and one of the physicians treating her son. The situation with the boy was presented as a background item, a form of stress which was viewed as a contributing factor to the marital conflict. Both Mr. and Mrs. G. focused on her infatuation with the physician as being the cause of their difficulties.

As treatment ensued, a different picture emerged. Both Mr. and Mrs. G. denied the full extent of their feelings about the boy's near death experience and subsequent difficult recovery. Yet their experience was clearly traumatic for the entire family. For over a year, they lived with uncertainty about his chances of survival. For two years, their lives were dominated by his care. They were required to maintain an environment as nearly sterile as possible. They had to perform around-the-clock procedures that regularly interrupted their sleep. As this routine developed, they fell into consistent roles. Mr. G. made himself into an expert on the medical procedures. He would come home in the evening and evaluate his wife's handling of the procedures during the day. She lived in fear of his criticism.

At the same time, Mr. G. became more demanding with the older boy, whose natural activities around the home threatened their ability to maintain the sterile environment. Mrs. G. made herself the champion of the older boy. She felt Mr. G. was harsh with the older boy and was ignoring his need for a warmer relationship with his father. She felt the boy was suffering as a result of it. The older boy became somewhat withdrawn, while the younger boy was viewed as heroic. Additionally, Mrs. G. quit sharing her emotional needs with her husband and found the physician to be a more understanding and caring listener.

Structure

From a structural family systems perspective, several key elements changed as a result of the crisis with the younger son.

1 The balance of power between the parents shifted. When Mr. G. put himself in the position of critiquing Mrs. G.'s care of the boy, he put himself on a different level from her. Their ability to function as partners was severely compromised by this.

2 The roles changed. Prior to the son's surgeries, both parents had been successful workers and relatively equal in their caretaking of the boys. After the surgeries, Mrs. G. gave up her job and focused on the home. She became the primary nurturer of the older boy, and Mr. G. became the primary disciplinarian of the older boy.

3 There was a major shift in the pattern of support and nurturance in the family. Mr. G withdrew his support of the older boy, and Mrs. G increased hers.

Affection between Mr. and Mrs. G came to a halt. Mrs. G began to direct her need for support outside of the family.

4 There was a major shift in the boundaries in the family. The boundary between husband and wife became rigid, while the boundary between mother and the older boy became more enmeshed. Mr. G. felt himself to be less a member of the family, even while he asserted more authority within the group.

5 A new triangle was established. The shift in the marital relationship was justified by the involvement of the younger son.

Rules

The rules changed. All of the above structural changes were accompanied by different rules. Mother was no longer to be obeyed on an equal level with father. The older boy was expected to show more self-control than before the trauma. It was not permissible for mother to challenge father. The structure was upheld through increased blaming and criticism. In many respects, they had become a different family, operating according to a very different set of rules.

Emotion

It is in the arena of emotionality and support that this family most clearly demonstrates the relationship between exposure to trauma and the functioning of an intact group. Prior to their son's surgeries, Mr. and Mrs. G. functioned relatively well as marital partners. They were a stable group joined in the shared task of caring for their family, i.e., themselves and their children. They were able to support each other and get the essential job done. This is not to say that they were free of problems. When they examined their earlier relationship, they were able to see glimmerings of many of the issues that flared into major problems. Mr. G. always had some tendency to become overly task-focused and unempathic to his effect on others. Mrs. G. always had some tendencies to feel bad about herself when criticized and to withdraw rather than confront. Indeed, most of the traits that they objected to in each other were present prior to the trauma. But they had found a way to live with these issues and function effectively as parents and marital partners.

The trauma disrupted their previous state of equilibrium. Warmth disappeared within the couple and Mr. G. was much less warm with the older boy. The control also changed radically, and it was applied inconsistently as Mr. and Mrs. G. began to struggle for control by undermining each other with the boys. The result was that the provision of emotional support was seriously damaged within the family.

Treatment

Treatment was initially sought to resolve the marital conflict. As the specific problems were discussed, the therapist helped the couple agree on the need to recover consistent caretaking of the family. An early obstacle was the family perception, propagated primarily by Mr. G., that the younger son would die if his physical treatment was handled in anything other than the compulsively perfectionistic style defined by Mr. G. These beliefs were challenged directly and Mr. G. was required to step back some and allow Mrs. G. to demonstrate her competence. This pattern was enacted in the transactions in the sessions, in which he would correct her and dominate the discussions. The therapist interrupted this communication pattern in the sessions and talked with the couple about the same patterns at home. As Mrs. G. was encouraged to become more of an equal partner in the physical care and decision-making at home, Mr. G. was encouraged to become more involved in the nurturing of the older son.

It was some time into the therapy before feelings of safety developed enough that each parent could dare to express the fear that had dominated his or her internal life for the past two years. Mr. G. was gradually able to see how he had, in fact, distanced from both of his children because of his fear of losing them. The younger son's physical condition was a constant reminder to Mr. G. and he had dealt with this by focusing on the boy's physical care and blinding himself to the child's emotional needs. At the same time, Mrs. G. had fallen into old patterns of incompetence which she had manifested in her family of origin years earlier. Her only means of fighting back was to treat Mr. G. as though he was not really a member of the family; in her mind, she made him disappear.

The older boy's withdrawal dissipated in correlation with his father's efforts to reach out to him. The family structure returned to a more balanced and effective arrangement, however, it was quite some time before the marital relationship regained its warmth and safety. In time, the entire family again came to operate as a supportive, cohesive group.

CONCLUSION

This chapter has focused on the family as a primary form of group treatment for PTSD. The treatment is focused on: (a) facilitating the family's support of the traumatized member, (b) helping the other members of the family who are affected by the traumatized member, and (c) helping the entire family function as an effective team in dealing with traumatic stressors. The therapist helps both the family group to take care of its members and the members to take care of their family group.

As in other forms of group treatment with PTSD, a primary task of the therapist is to attend to the group members' difficulties with the traumatic affect and cognitions (Catherall & Shelton, 1996). Because families are intact groups with a history, the treatment is likely to encounter additional problems, such as the stirring of old injuries and conflicts. But the thrust of treatment is fundamentally the same as in other psychotherapeutic groups, the therapist works to facilitate the group process and the healing properties of caring relationships. Perhaps the major difference between family work and a psychotherapy group is that families have the strongest bonds and, therefore, the greatest potential for healing.

REFERENCES

Ackerman, N. W. (1937). The family as a social and emotional unit. *Bulletin of the Kansas Mental Hygiene Society, 12*(2).

Ackerman, N. W. (1954). Interpersonal disturbances in the family: Some unresolved problems in psychotherapy. *Psychiatry, 17,* 359–368.

Ackerman, N. W., & Behrens, M. L. (1956). A study of family diagnosis. *American Journal of Orthopsychiatry, 26,* 66-78.

Catherall, D. R. (1989). Differentiating intervention strategies for primary and secondary trauma in post-traumatic stress disorder: The example of Vietnam veterans. *Journal of Traumatic Stress, 2*(3), 289–304.

Catherall, D. R. (1991). Aggression and projective identification in the treatment of victims. *Psychotherapy* (Special Issue: Psychotherapy with Victims), *28*(1), 145–149.

Catherall, D. R. (1992). *Back from the brink: A family guide to overcoming traumatic stress.* New York: Bantam.

Catherall, D. R. (1995). Coping with secondary traumatic stress: The importance of the therapist's professional peer group. In B. H. Stamm (Ed.), *Secondary traumatic stress: Self-care issues for clinicians, researchers, and educators* (pp. 80–92). Lutherville, MD: Sidran.

Catherall, D. R. (1998). Treating traumatized families. In C. R. Figley (Ed.), *Burnout in families: The systemic costs of caring* (pp. 185–212). St. Lucie Press Innovations in Psychology Book Series.

Catherall, D. R., & Shelton, R. B. (1996). Men's groups for post-traumatic stress disorder and the role of shame. In M. P. Andronico (Ed.), *Men in groups: Insights, interventions, psychoeducational work* (pp. 323–337). Washington, DC: American Psychological Association.

Cusinato, M. (1998). Parenting styles and psychopathology. In L. L'Abate (Ed.), *Family psychopathology: The relational roots of dysfunctional behavior* (pp. 158–179). New York: Guilford.

Danieli, Y. (1985). The treatment and prevention of long-term effects and intergenerational transmission of victimization: A lesson from Holocaust survivors and their children. In C. R. Figley (Ed.), *Trauma and its wake, volume I: The study and treatment of post-traumatic stress disorder* (pp. 295–313). New York: Brunner/Mazel.

Figley, C. R. (1989). *Helping traumatized families.* San Francisco: Jossey-Bass.

Figley, C. R. (1995). *Compassion fatigue: Coping with secondary traumatic stress disorder in those who treat the traumatized.* New York: Brunner/Mazel.

Figley, C. R. (1998). Introduction. In C. R. Figley (Ed.), *Burnout in families: The systemic costs of caring.* St. Lucie Press Innovations in Psychology Book Series.

Frank, J. (1961). *Persuasion and healing.* Baltimore: Johns Hopkins University Press.

Free, K., Alechina, I., & Zahn-Waxler, C. (1996). Affective language between depressed mothers and their children: The potential impact of psychotherapy. *Journal of the American Academy of Child and Adolescent Psychiatry, 35,* 783–790.

Gottman, J. M., Katz, L. F., & Hooven, C. (1996). Parental meta-emotion philosophy and the emotional life of families: Theoretical models and preliminary data. *Journal of Family Psychology, 10,* 243–268.

Greening, L., & Dollinger, S. J. (1992). Illusions (and shattered illusions) of invulnerability: Adolescents in natural disaster. *Journal of Traumatic Stress, 5*(1), 63–76.

Haley, J. (1963). *Strategies of psychotherapy.* New York: Grune & Stratton.

Herman, J. L. (1992). *Trauma and recovery.* New York: Basic Books.

Hinde, R. A. (1995). A suggested structure for a science of relationship. *Personal Relationships, 2,* 1–15.

Jackson, D. D. (1957). The question of family homeostasis. *The Psychiatric Quarterly Supplement, 31,* 79–90.

Jackson, D. D. (1965). Family rules: The marital quid pro quo. *Archives of General Psychiatry, 12,* 589–594.

Jaques, E. (1955). Social systems as defense against persecutory and depressive anxiety. In M. Klein (Ed.), *New directions in psychoanalysis.* New York: Basic Books.

Lindy, J. (1985). The trauma membrane and other clinical concepts derived from psychotherapeutic work with survivors of natural disasters. *Psychiatric Annals, 15*(3), 153–160.

Lindy, J. (1986). An outline for the psychoanalytic psychotherapy of post-traumatic stress disorder. In C. R. Figley (Ed.), *Trauma and its wake, volume II: Traumatic stress theory, research, and intervention* (pp. 195–212). New York: Brunner/Mazel.

Loukas, A., Twitchell, G. R., Piejak, L. A., Fitzgerald, H. E., & Zucker, R. A. (1998). The family as a unity of interacting personalities. In L. L'Abate (Ed.), *Family psychopathology: The relational roots of dysfunctional behavior* (pp. 35–59). New York: Guilford.

McCann, I. L., & Pearlman, L. A. (1990). Vicarious traumatization: A framework for understanding the psychological effects of working with victims. *Journal of Traumatic Stress, 3*(1), 131–150.

McCubbin, H. I., & Figley, C. R. (1983). Bridging normative and catastrophic family stress. In H. I. McCubbin & C. R. Figley (Eds.), *Stress and the family: Vol. 1. Coping with normative transitions* (pp. 218–228). New York: Brunner/Mazel.

Minuchin, S. (1974). *Families and family therapy.* Cambridge, MA: Harvard University Press.

Minuchin, S. (1979). Constructing a therapeutic reality. In E. Kaufman & P.N. Kaufman (Eds.), *Family therapy of drug and alcohol abuse.* New York: Gardner Press.

Nathanson, D. L. (1992). *Shame and pride: Affect, sex, and the birth of the self.* New York: Norton.

Ochberg, F. M. (1991). Post-traumatic therapy. *Psychotherapy* (Special Issue: Psychotherapy with Victims), *28*(1), 5–15.

Paul, N. L., & Grosser, G. H. (1965). Operational mourning and its role in conjoint family therapy. *Community Mental Health Journal, 1,* 339–345.

Scabini, E., & Cigoli, V. (1998). The role of theory in the study of family psychopathology. In L. L'Abate (Ed.), *Family psychopathology: The relational roots of dysfunctional behavior* (pp. 13–34). New York: Guilford.

Singer, M. T., & Wynne, L. C. (1965). Thought disorder and family relations of schizophrenics: III. Methodology using projective techniques. *Archives of General Psychiatry, 12,* 187–200.

Stiver, I. P. (1990a). *Dysfunctional families and wounded relationships—Part I.* Work in progress. Wellesley, MA: Stone Center Working Paper Series.

Stiver, I. P. (1990b). *Dysfunctional families and wounded relationships—Part II.* Work in progress. Wellesley, MA: Stone Center Working Paper Series.

Wagner, B. M., & Reiss, D. (1995). Family systems and developmental psychopathology: Courtship, marriage, or divorce? In D. Cicchetti & D. J. Cohen (Eds.), *Developmental psychopathology, Volume 1. Theory and methods* (pp. 696–730). New York: Wiley.

Watzlawick, P., Beavin, J. H., & Jackson, D. D. (1967). *Pragmatics of human communication.* New York: Norton.

Yalom, I. D. (1985). *The theory and practice of group psychotherapy,* Third edition. New York: Basic Books.

Chapter 3

Group Treatment of Sexual Assault Survivors

Kathleen M. Chard, Patricia A. Resick, and Janice J. Wertz

Epidemiological studies have found that 13% to 22% (Kilpatrick et al., 1992; Koss, Gidycz,& Wisniewski, 1987) of adult women living in the United States have been raped. This act of interpersonal violence can have long term ramifications including, anxiety, depression, sexual dysfunction, low self-esteem, and more commonly, symptoms of post-traumatic stress disorder (PTSD). In fact, a longitudinal study (Rothbaum, Foa, Riggs, Murdock, & Walsh, 1992) showed that 47% of rape victims met the criteria for PTSD three months after the assault and at a nine-month follow-up.

These statistics clearly indicate that a significant number of individuals may be trying to manage trauma-related symptoms. Until recently, victims seeking group therapy were treated with either supportive or psychodynamic group interventions (e.g., Cryer & Beutler, 1980; Roth, Dye, & Leibowitz, 1988). In the early 1980's cognitive-behavioral researchers, utilizing controlled studies, began applying learning and information processing theories to the understanding of symptom response and the treatment of assault victims (Foa, Rothbaum, & Steketee, 1993; Resick & Schnicke, 1990). Many of these studies utilized individual therapy interventions, such as cognitive-behavioral therapy (Frank et al., 1988), stress inoculation training (Resick, Jordan, Girelli, Hutter, & Marhoefer-Dvorak, 1988), prolonged exposure (Foa, Rothbaum, Riggs, & Murdock, 1991; Foa, Jaycox, Meadows, Hembree, & Dancu, 1996), and cognitive processing therapy (Resick, Nishith, & Astin, 1996; Resick & Schnicke, 1993). Due to fiscal and time demands, there has also been a recent emphasis on cognitive-behavioral group interventions (e.g., Resick et al., 1988).

This chapter will provide the following information with regard to treating sexual assault victims using group therapy: (a) a discussion of the existing empirically-based group therapy approaches, along with outcome results from the research, (b) an outline of the principles and techniques of Cognitive Processing Therapy (CPT), an empirically-based treatment approach specifically designed to address symptoms commonly seen in rape victims, and (c) suggestions of possible contraindications for utilizing CPT and group treatments with rape victims in general.

EMPIRICAL RESEARCH

Empirical research focusing on group therapy with sexual assault victims is relatively sparse. Of those studies that have been conducted, some are methodologically limited by small sample sizes, no pre- and posttreatment data, lack of a specific treatment outline or manual, no use of a control group, and/or no comparison with other treatment approaches. In addition, few of these studies have focused on PTSD, the disorder most often associated with rape victims. The following section will review existing group treatments, with a brief discussion of the therapy format and research findings.

Stress Inoculation Training

Stress Inoculation Training (SIT) was developed by Meichenbaum (1985) and was adapted by Kilpatrick and colleagues (Kilpatrick, Veronen, & Resick, 1982; Kilpatrick & Amick, 1985) for use with rape survivors. Using a social learning framework, the main purpose of SIT is to provide clients with coping skills to deal with everyday life stressors, and, more specifically, to moderate fear and anxiety. SIT is made up of several phases that can be used within group or individual therapy. The first phase is primarily educational, in which clients are given a social learning explanation of their response to trauma. After the educational phase, the therapist provides coping skills training, giving clients a definition, rationale, and explanation of various coping skills. Skills typically taught in the groups include muscle relaxation, controlled breathing, covert modeling, role-playing, thought stopping, and guided self-dialogue.

Resick et al. (1988) compared group formats of SIT (N = 12), assertion training (N = 13), and supportive psychotherapy (N = 12) (including an information/education phase) to a wait-list control group in a six-week, two hours per week, format. Results indicate that all three of the group treatments were more effective than the control group in producing lasting improvements, particularly with regard to fear and anxiety. However, there were no statistically significant differences among the treatment groups. At a six-month follow-up, the improvements remained for the rape-related fears, but not for depression, self-esteem, and social fears.

Supportive/Psychotherapy Groups

Supportive group treatments for rape victims, similar to support groups in general, provide key aspects to the members. Group members share their experiences and provide emotional support, which generally results in a decrease in isolation when the victim discovers there are others who have experienced a similar trauma. Having a common bond with other individuals also tends to provide validation and normalization of the common reactions associated with rape. Support groups also allow members to relate similar issues and to share coping methods and insights. By relating in a group format, members can witness other individuals at different points in the recovery process and can recognize their progress, as well as envision the recovery that is possible.

Cryer and Beutler (1980) conducted a ten-week, 1½ hours per week, support group with nine women. All symptoms, including anxiety were decreased significantly. Limitations of the study included the lack of a comparison or control group and the absence of a PTSD measure. In addition, the absence of a specific format within the group makes replication of the study and the treatment difficult.

Roth, Dye, and Leibowitz (1988) compared a year long psychotherapy group for rape victims (N=7) with a control group (N=6). Treatment consisted of a total of 47 sessions, each of which lasted an average of 2½ hours. All of the members of the treatment group were in individual therapy at some point during treatment. The group therapy was based on Horowitz's (1976) model of psychological response and offered supportive interactions between group members and coleaders. By the 20th session, treatment group participants showed an improvement in rape-related fears, adjustment, and intrusive symptoms. Improvements on depression scores were displayed by the 28th session. The reduction of fear, improvement of depression, and intrusion relief was maintained at a six month follow-up. Interestingly, both treatment and control subjects showed improvement in PTSD symptoms from the first to the second assessment points.

Cognitive Processing Therapy

Cognitive Processing Therapy (CPT) was developed as a specific treatment package tailored to the needs of rape victims with symptoms of depression, PTSD, and cognitive distortions (Resick & Schnicke, 1993). Combining elements of Beck's Cognitive Behavior Therapy with procedures derived from information processing theories, CPT can be implemented in either a group or individual format.

Resick and Schnicke (1992) compared CPT group treatment (N = 19) consisting of twelve 1½ hour sessions to a wait-list control group (N = 20). Significant improvements were reported for CPT participants from pre- to posttreatment on both PTSD and depression measures and improvements were maintained over a six-month period following treatment. The control group, however, did not display significant changes between the two assessment periods.

PRINCIPLES AND TECHNIQUES OF GROUP WORK WITH RAPE VICTIMS

Therapeutic Rationale

As noted above, there are several group treatments for rape survivors available for use by practitioners. Yet, within the past several years, emphasis has been placed on identifying a theory-based treatment that addresses the etiology and manifestation of the symptoms associated with sexual assault. In addition, practitioners are becoming increasingly interested in treatments that have reduced symptoms of PTSD and depression. Finally, with the increasing demands of managed care, practitioners are seeking short-term, manualized treatments with demonstrated efficacy. In a meta-analysis conducted by Chard (1994), cognitive interventions were found to be superior to cognitive-behavior, supportive, and psychodynamic interventions for the reduction of symptoms related to sexual assault. To date, CPT is the only empirically-based, manualized, short-term, cognitive, group treatment available for practitioners who work with sexual assault survivors. For descriptive purposes, the rest of the chapter will focus on factors affecting the implementation of CPT in a group format.

Client Selection/Assessment

The initial factor in screening for group members is to identify sexual assault in a client's history. Frequently, unless they are asked directly, rape victims will not disclose that they have been assaulted. Nondisclosure is common and is in keeping with the client's pattern of avoiding trauma-related stimuli. Often when rape victims seek treatment, they do not identify their psychological symptoms as being trauma-related. Further, due to their assimilation of the event, many sexual assault victims do not label their experience as rape, because they may fear disbelief or blame from anyone they tell. To facilitate the identification and selection of group members, we recommend the use of both structured clinical interviews and psychometric instruments. We assess clients before, after, and sometimes during treatment, even when they are not participating in one of our research studies. The information provided in the assessment is invaluable for gauging the client's level of distress and identifying the most elevated PTSD symptoms, particularly if the client has higher levels of reexperiencing and lower levels of avoidance. This pattern indicates that the client is continuing to process the event at some level and is not actively avoiding her thoughts and feelings. If instead the client is high on avoidance and low on intrusion, she may be engaging in avoidant coping behaviors that will make her more resistant to therapy. In this situation, the therapist will need to help the client focus on her thoughts and feelings related to the rape and other situations.

Often in the assessment we find clients who have high levels of depressive symptomatology as well as PTSD. This may indicate a more pervasive problem of cognitive-distortions, lower self-esteem, and more feelings of hopelessness. The ongoing assessment can monitor these thoughts and feelings, especially as the client goes though the difficult process of writing about the assault. This midtreatment assessment also allows the client and therapist to see gains that have been made, especially when the client becomes stuck on one area. Although our research assessment battery is quite lengthy, we recommend the following instruments for individual clients: Beck Depression Inventory (BDI; Beck, Ward, Mendelson, Mock & Erbaugh, 1961), PTSD Symptom Scale (PSS-SR; Resick, Falsetti, Resnick & Kilpatrick, 1991), and the Clinician Administered PTSD Scale (CAPS; Blake et al, 1990).

Researchers (Koss & Harvey, 1991; McCann & Pearlman, 1990) have noted that there are some clients who are poor candidates for group therapy. These include clients who have substance dependence problems, those who are suicidal, clients with borderline personality disorder and who are currently self-mutilating, clients who have never talked about the trauma before, or those who have very fragmented memories of the trauma. We refer these clients into individual therapy until they become more stabilized, at which time they may be rescreened for the group. Because CPT is a structured, time-limited treatment, it would be very difficult to offer this treatment in an inpatient setting with rotating admissions, and abbreviated lengths of stay. In addition, clients in an inpatient facility may not be stable enough to address their assault to the degree that may be required for successful alleviation of symptoms.

Cognitive Processing Therapy Treatment

Cognitive Processing Therapy (CPT) is a 12-session, structured treatment program that can be used in either an individual or group setting. Group treatment is conducted in weekly 90-minute sessions, preferably with coleaders. Treatment is based on an information processing model of PTSD and combines components of exposure-based therapies with cognitive restructuring elements of cognitive therapy. The cognitive portion of the therapy challenges specific cognitions that are most likely to have been disrupted by the trauma. Following is a brief description of the 12-session group treatment format of CPT.

Session 1: Introduction and Education Phase   The overall objectives of the first session are to provide information about the development of PTSD and to outline the course of treatment. Group members are informed that the treatment is fairly structured and will involve homework, with each assignment building upon the last. As such, compliance in attending sessions and completing homework is emphasized.

In explaining why PTSD symptoms develop, rape is described as schema-discrepant, i.e., most women do not have preexisting schemas with which to organize the event. Instead, a woman may alter her memories or interpretation of the event to fit current dysfunctional beliefs (assimilation). Examples of assimilation are when a woman blames herself for not preventing a rape or distorts the event so as not to label it as rape. Accommodation, which is a goal of CPT, occurs when a woman changes her beliefs in order to organize the experience cognitively (e.g., "I was raped by someone I knew."). Some women, however, tend to overaccommodate (e.g., "No man can be trusted."), which is also disruptive and therefore challenged in CPT.

In addition to accommodation, other therapy goals include having individuals experience their feelings about the event and helping them to recognize and modify thoughts that are interfering with recovery. These problematic beliefs, known as "stuck points," are conflicts between prior beliefs and the rape, or they involve prior dysfunctional beliefs that are confirmed by the rape. In the first session, a handout is provided to group members that describes and provides examples of stuck points (Resick & Schnicke, 1993). One example of a stuck point might be if an individual previously believed she could not be raped by someone she knew and then was raped by an acquaintance.

For homework, each group member is to write at least one page on what it means to have been raped. Individuals are to focus on how the rape affected their belief system about themselves, others, and the world in connection to five core areas: safety, trust, power/control, esteem, and intimacy.

Session 2: The Meaning of the Event   The two main purposes of the second group session include: (a) discussing the meaning of the rape and looking for stuck points, and (b) helping the group members to begin to label their emotions, to recognize their thoughts, and to look at the connection between their thoughts and feelings (Calhoun & Resick, 1993).

The group is initiated by reviewing the homework and having clients share their reactions to the assignment. Often, stuck points will be identified and the process of addressing these can be initiated. Next, the leaders facilitate a discussion of four basic emotional responses (mad, sad, glad, and scared) and describe how interpretations and self-statements affect feelings. To increase awareness about the connection between an event and subsequent thoughts, feelings, and behaviors, homework involves having members complete A-B-C sheets (i.e., Activating Event, Beliefs, Consequences) (see Appendix A). Members are asked to complete at least one sheet in connection with their thoughts about the rape and other sheets for everyday events. At the end of this session, the meaning-of-the-event statements are collected and held until the final session.

Session 3: Identification of Thoughts and Feelings   The A-B-C sheets completed as homework are reviewed at the beginning of group. Each member is then asked to pick one event and to try different self-statements in order to modify her affective response. In reviewing the sheet completed about the rape, the members and group leaders attempt to identify stuck points that resulted from the trauma.

Homework for the subsequent week is for each group member to write a detailed account of the rape and to include as many sensory details (sights, sounds, smells, and so on), thoughts, and feelings as she can recall. Members are also instructed to read the entire account to themselves at least once prior to the next session, but preferably daily. If a group member has been raped more than once, she is asked to write about the most traumatic event first.

Session 4: Remembering the Rape   Sessions 4 and 5 constitute the exposure component of CPT (Resick & Schnicke, 1992). The purpose is to subject each individual to the details of the rape that she has avoided and to allow her emotions to be expressed and extinguished. Group members discuss their reactions to the homework and focus on the thoughts they had and feelings they experienced while performing the assignment. However, to avoid secondary traumatization, group members are never asked to describe the rape in detail to other group members.

Written accounts are collected and reviewed by the therapists in order to provide members with additional assistance in identifying stuck points. Places where the client stopped writing (as indicated by her drawing a line) are noted because they may signal a place of particular difficulty. The therapist also reads each account to determine if it contains expressed emotion. Recounting a rape without much emotion may indicate a client fears a loss of control or the possibility of being overwhelmed by her feelings.

When reviewing each account, the therapist also focuses on which parts of the event an individual is unable to remember. Dissociative reactions and the most frightening parts of the experience may not be remembered initially. Difficult memories often signal incomplete processing and therefore stuck points that interfere with adaptive accommodation. As cognitive conflicts are resolved, the majority of group members are able to recover most memories and to experience their emotions.

For homework, group participants are asked to write the entire account of their rape again and to add more sensory details, thoughts, and feelings. In parentheses they are to indicate the thoughts and feelings they experience while writing. The account is to be read daily prior to the next session.

Session 5: Identification of Stuck Points   Again the session is initiated by obtaining members' reactions to their homework assignment. Within this discussion, individuals are asked to express the differences and similarities between how they felt at the time of the rape and how they felt when writing the written account. They are also asked to compare their feelings when writing and reading about the rape the second time in comparison to the first. If an individual allowed herself to experience her emotions with the initial writing, the intensity will most likely have decreased with the second exercise. The therapists can cite this to point out how the intensity of emotion will decrease over time. On the other hand, the individual may experience a temporary increase in the intensity of her emotions if she avoided her feelings during the first assignment.

A list of *Challenging Questions* (Resick & Schnicke, 1993, adapted from Beck and Emery, 1985) (see Appendix B) is introduced during this session to help group members confront maladaptive self-statements and stuck points. Individuals write down a belief they wish to challenge (e.g., "Because I didn't fight back, it was my fault that I was raped") and then answer a set of 12 questions (e.g., What is the evidence for and against this idea? Are you taking selected examples out of context?). As homework, each member chooses several stuck points and answers the challenging questions in connection with each belief. In addition, if an individual experienced more than one rape, she is instructed to begin writing in detail about the second most traumatic event.

Session 6: Challenging Questions   The session begins by discussing the group members' challenging questions sheets. As one individual provides her responses, the therapists and other group members can help her analyze and confront the belief. At this point in the therapeutic process, stuck points often surround the themes of self-blame and beliefs that the situation could have been handled differently. For resolution, it is important that the leaders help members identify underlying attributions and conflicting cognitions in connection with these issues.

In the latter part of the session, Beck's faulty thinking patterns (e.g., overgeneralization and mind reading) are introduced and a *Faulty Thinking Patterns* handout with examples is provided (see Appendix C). For homework, each member is asked to consider new stuck points as well as those stuck points already discussed in order to identify how they fit with the faulty thinking patterns listed on the handout. Group participants are also asked to look for specific ways their reactions to the rape may have been affected by these habitual thinking patterns.

Session 7: Faulty Thinking Patterns   In this session, the faulty thinking patterns are discussed in terms of how they become automatic and how they can lead to negative feelings and self-defeating behaviors (for example, limiting social activities and avoiding meeting people after concluding that the world is not safe). After reviewing the homework, the *Challenging Beliefs Worksheet* (Resick & Schnicke, 1993; adapted from Beck & Emery, 1985, p. 205) (see Appendix D) is introduced to assist members in further confronting and changing faulty cognitions. Individuals are instructed to identify and rate (from 0% to 100%) their emotional reaction and to describe the situation that led to the reaction. They also write down and rate their automatic thinking and then use the *Challenging Questions* and *Faulty Thinking Patterns* handouts to examine their thoughts. The individuals' alternative thoughts as well what they feel are the worst consequences that could realistically occur are also recorded. Finally, individuals are instructed to evaluate the outcome of this process by reevaluating their automatic thoughts and emotional reaction.

During the remainder of the session, the therapists instruct the group members that five life themes (safety, trust, power/control, esteem, and intimacy) may be significantly affected by rape and these topics will be the focus of the next five sessions. The topic of safety is introduced in a handout noting how an individual's beliefs about safety could be either disrupted or confirmed by a rape. Homework for Sessions 7 through 11 involves asking group members to use the *Challenging Beliefs Worksheets* to confront stuck points. Individuals are asked to pay particular attention to that week's topic in case it proves to be an issue in need of additional processing.

Session 8: Safety Issues   The session starts by reviewing the homework and determining how successful group members were in challenging cognitions related to safety issues. Often when clients first complete the *Challenging Beliefs Worksheets*, their cognitions are so entrenched that they have a difficult time taking other perspectives and providing alternative thoughts.

Safety is viewed with regard to the relative safety of others and to personal safety in terms of a woman's ability to protect herself. Part of the discussion focuses on how negative beliefs about safety can elicit anxiety and subsequent avoidance behavior. For group members who have safety issues, there is often a need to focus on the probability of a rape occurring and to remind individuals that in the course of everyday living, rape is relatively rare. After a rape, however, victims often behave as though it is an event of extremely high probability. Trust, an issue often related to safety, is introduced in the later part of the session as the second module (Resick & Schnicke, 1993) and again a handout is provided.

Session 9: Trust Issues   The challenging beliefs homework is reviewed, focusing on trust issues. Prior experiences in the development of positive or negative beliefs concerning one's own judgment or trust in others are discussed in terms of how a rape may serve to destroy or confirm these prior beliefs. For individuals who were raped by an acquaintance, trust can be of particular importance because thoughts of betrayal and doubt in one's own judgment are often prominent.

Resolution of trust issues is achieved by helping members realize that trust in self and others is not an all-or-nothing experience. An individual can still trust her judgment even though it is not perfect. And, although some people may be untrustworthy, others can be trusted. Rather than starting from a position of complete trust or complete distrust, clients are advised to begin from a middle position (no information), and are told that interactions with a person will provide information about trust. The therapists can also empathize by indicating that developing trust involves risk and that the process can be frightening. A rape victim is often overly suspicious as a means of self-protection. However, her suspicion may result in feeling isolated and alienated because of missed opportunities for developing new relationships that could provide intimacy and support. Brainstorming may be necessary to identify safety precautions that can be taken while developing trust in new relationships.

The third module, power and control (Resick & Schnicke, 1993) is introduced toward the end of the ninth session. Additional explanation is provided in a handout given to the clients.

Session 10: Power and Control Issues   The session is initiated by reviewing the members' attempts at changing cognitions regarding power and control, again using the *Challenging Beliefs Worksheet*. Self-power is an individual's belief that she can meet challenges and solve problems. Because the rape was out of her control, a rape victim may overcompensate and attempt complete control of other situations and her own emotions. If not experiencing complete control, she may feel as though she is completely out of control, which again represents either-or thinking. Power in relation to others revolves around beliefs that one can control future outcomes in interpersonal relationships, that one has power even when relating to powerful others, or that others have power or control over you. Once again, prior experiences affect the individual's beliefs, and a rape can confirm negative or disrupt positive cognitions with regard to power and control. Resolution involves helping group members strike a balance between wanting complete control versus feeling completely powerless. The group leaders can help the members to see that no one has complete control over all situations or other people, nor are they completely helpless.

Women frequently experience anger at this point in therapy, and these feelings can frighten them. Societal messages have discouraged women from expressing anger, and individuals may fear losing control or becoming aggressive if they express their emotional response. The therapists can help validate group members' anger as a legitimate reaction to having power and control taken from them during the rape and can reassure them that experiencing anger does not have to lead to aggression.

The remaining group time is devoted to discussing the esteem module and to reviewing an *Identifying Assumptions Sheet* (Beck & Emery, 1985) (see Appendix E). This sheet lists basic assumptions in three areas (acceptance, competence, and control) and each individual is asked to identify those statements she believes to be true of her. Examples of the common assumptions are "I'm nothing unless I'm loved," "I have to be somebody," and "I can't ask for help." The group leaders then explain why the common assumptions are faulty and extreme and how they can lead to depression. In addition to the standard homework, group members are asked to practice giving and receiving compliments and to do unconditionally at least one nice thing for themselves every day.

Session 11: Esteem Issues   Group members discuss the success of their efforts to give and receive compliments and to perform self-nurturing activities. They are also encouraged to continue these practices. When group members review their worksheets, a frequently encountered stuck point related to self-esteem is the belief that one is somehow damaged because she has been raped. This belief reflects faulty thinking, such as overgeneralization, mind reading and drawing conclusions, or all three.

Regarding esteem for others, it is not uncommon for some group members to overgeneralize their disregard for the rapist to an entire group. Certain beliefs may be generalized to all males, to a particular race or social class, or even to a profession. Furthermore, a rape victim will often have a heightened awareness of the media's reports of crime. It may appear as though crime is rampant and that all people are bad. When overgeneralization like this occurs, it is important to help the group member identify exceptions to her beliefs and if necessary, provide her with statistical information. Group members should be reminded that on a daily basis, the majority of people are not involved in a crime as either the victim or the assailant. Esteem issues can be resolved by helping individuals realize that bad things can happen to good people, that judging character is difficult and takes time, and that all people make mistakes at some time. The therapist can also point out that, in most cases, it is not a matter of a mistake or faulty judgment by the victim, but a surprising betrayal on the part of the assailant.

Intimacy, the final module (Resick & Schnicke, 1993), is introduced concerning how it has been affected by the rape. In addition to the standard homework of completing the challenging beliefs worksheets, group members are asked to rewrite their first assignment on what it means to have been raped.

Session 12: Intimacy Issues and the Meaning of the Event   The final assignment is reviewed to identify stuck points and to change cognitions in order to enhance intimacy. Problems with self-intimacy may be manifest in attempted self-soothing, yet often self-defeating behaviors such as abusing substances (food, alcohol, drugs, or tobacco) or through other external sources such as impulsive spending or promiscuous sex. The connection between being raped and harmful behaviors may not become apparent to the individual until she is in treatment. In addition, she may not have been aware of soothing alternatives. However, with CPT treatment, she learns to use worksheets to identify her thinking associated with anxious arousal. She can practice calming herself with more adaptive self-statements and behaviors instead of falling back on self-defeating habits.

Intimacy with others, i.e., closeness with family and friends and sexual intimacy, are frequently affected by rape. Social withdrawal from others allows many rape survivors to feel safer and to avoid possible rejection and blame, but they may also end up feeling isolated and alone. Sexual intimacy may trigger frightening memories and may be difficult because of the level of trust and vulnerability required. Resolving intimacy and trust issues requires that group members monitor and challenge their cognitions, take manageable risks, and communicate with others whom they feel have let them down. Talking with others allows a rape survivor to determine if these people can meet her needs or if the relationship needs to be limited or dissolved.

Group members also discuss their reactions to writing about the meaning of the rape a second time and compare this assignment to the first time they performed this exercise. Members are encouraged to look for how their beliefs have changed and to identify faulty thinking that may need additional intervention. Most group members notice significant changes, particularly in terms of increased self-understanding and finding some positive meaning from the event (e.g., the benefits of the therapy that resulted from the rape). Finally, the rest of the session is devoted to reviewing skills and progress, emphasizing the need for continuing the skills developed, and identifying future goals and social support systems. This focus on the future is done, in part, to prevent relapse and to encourage clients to continue to apply the techniques they have learned to upcoming challenges.

Therapists' Roles

With CPT, the therapists' primary roles are to structure the group sessions, challenge faulty cognitions, and disseminate information as discussed in the foregoing section. Although it is possible for one therapist to run a group, having coleaders provides a number of benefits. While one leader is presenting new material or working more directly with one member, the other therapist can observe group process and bring these observations into the discussion. In addition, pragmatically it is difficult for one therapist to review all of the homework and respond to written assignments in a thorough manner.

CONTRAINDICATIONS

In addition to numerous advantages that group therapy offers rape survivors, there are also several drawbacks. As discussed earlier, care should be taken when selecting group members because certain individuals are poor candidates. A thorough assessment and screening can help to eliminate or reduce a number of potential problems. McCann and Pearlman (1990) suggest that clients with severe PTSD should receive simultaneous individual and group treatment because therapy may elicit strong affect and memories that can be experienced as overwhelming and individual therapy can offset these strong reactions. However, receiving both forms of therapy at the same time can be confusing for the client, especially if the therapists have different theoretical orientations (Calhoun & Resick, 1994). It is often better for the client to be solely in individual therapy or to be in individual treatment long enough for her to develop coping skills that enable her to benefit from group treatment.

One of the most common problems encountered in performing CPT group therapy is incomplete homework (Resick & Schnicke, 1993). Not completing homework most often reflects avoidance. Some clients avoid material because it is experienced as too emotionally laden and the individual is afraid of being overwhelmed by her thoughts, feelings, and memories. This belief can be addressed as a stuck point that needs to be challenged in order for the individual to benefit from the CPT model. However, this confrontation may be more difficult to do in a group setting.

On occasion, group members have difficulty completing homework because the act of writing down their experiences makes the event and their reactions too real to manage. Denial can be especially strong in women who have not labeled their experience as rape. These clients' beliefs can be challenged by pointing out that their traumatic reactions, as indicated on pretreatment assessment measures, provide evidence that the event was a rape and is disrupting their life.

Some of the general disadvantages of group treatment also apply to CPT. Many of these potential problems can be addressed by attending to group dynamics and intervening at the group level. As mentioned previously, an advantage of having cotherapists is that while one therapist is presenting new material or facilitating the discussion, the other therapist can observe group process and address group dynamics.

One drawback of a group format is that less individual attention is available for each member. Furthermore, differences in personality styles and interpersonal conflicts are inherent in the group process. Group members who have a dominant communication style may cause other members to be slighted and may exacerbate the avoidance associated with rape. A group format may also make it difficult for individuals who are shy or for members who are reluctant to talk because they are avoiding the subject matter. Another potential problem with a group format is that certain members of the group may not get along and one or more may be ostracized. The ostracized members may not be given as much opportunity to talk or may not receive as much support from other group members. Estranged members will probably not find the group as helpful and may even feel harmed (Resick & Schnicke, 1993). If a member of the group is being sidelined, it is the responsibility of the therapists to bring the individual back into the group by addressing group process or by engaging them either through direct comments or in some other manner.

Secondary traumatization, a potential problem associated with other group treatments for rape survivors, is avoided with CPT. Secondary traumatization can occur when a group member is exposed to the accounts of other members. It is often very difficult for clients to integrate their own rape experiences, and hearing other stories of traumatization may impede treatment. Hearing other members' accounts may result in an individual focusing on others instead of herself and her own treatment goals (Resick & Schnicke, 1993). These potential problems are avoided by never asking group members to describe their rape experience in detail while in group.

CONCLUSION

As evidenced by the above discussion, there are both advantages and disadvantages (contraindications) to group treatment. The advantages include cost effectiveness, social support, normalization, universality, and participants challenging one another's faulty cognitions, thereby enhancing skill development. These advantages make group therapy a very appealing treatment choice for sexual assault survivors.

Unfortunately, there has been very little research on group therapy outcome, leaving clinicians with a limited number of empirically-based treatment options from which to choose. It is very important to conduct such research in order to establish efficacy of the various treatment models in the literature today. One of the problems with group research is that it is difficult to obtain enough clients at any one time for random assignment to treatment or wait-list conditions. One possible solution would be conducting multi-site research studies, involving several agencies. Also, given the managed care inclination toward group therapy, it is important to compare group versus individual treatment. While group treatment is cost effective in terms of therapist-client ratio, it will be important to determine if group is as efficacious as individual treatment.

REFERENCES

Beck, A. T., & Emery, G. (1985). *Anxiety disorders and phobias: A cognitive perspective.* New York: Basic Books.

Calhoun, K. S., & Atkeson, B. M. (1991). *Treatment of rape victims: Facilitating psychosocial adjustment.* New York: Pergamon Press.

Calhoun, K. S., & Resick, P. A. (1993). Post-traumatic stress disorder. In D. Barlow (Ed.), *Clinical handbook of psychological disorders: A step-by-step treatment manual* (pp. 48–98). New York: Guilford Press.

Chard, K. M. (1994). *A meta-analysis of post-traumatic stress disorder treatment outcome studies of sexually victimized women.* Unpublished doctoral dissertation, Indiana University, Bloomington.

Cryer, L., & Beutler, L. (1980). Group therapy: An alternative treatment approach for rape victims. *Journal of Sex and Marital Therapy, 6,* 40–46.

Foa, E. B., Jaycox, L. H., Meadows, E. A., Hembree, E., & Dancu, C. V. (1996). Preliminary efficacy of prolonged exposure (PE) vs. PE and cognitive restructuring for PTSD in female assault victims. In P. Resick (Chair), *Treating sexual assault/sexual abuse pathology: Recent findings.* Symposium conducted at the annual convention of the Association for Advancement of Behavior Therapy, New York.

Foa, E. B., Rothbaum, B. O., Riggs, D. S., & Murdock, T. B. (1991). Treatment of post-traumatic stress disorder in rape victims: A comparison between cognitive-behavioral procedures and counseling. *Journal of Consulting and Clinical Psychology, 59,* 715–723.

Foa, E. B., Rothbaum, B. O., & Steketee, G. S. (1993). Treatment of rape victims. *Journal of Interpersonal Violence, 8,* 256–276.

Frank, E., Anderson, B., Stewart, B. D., Dancu, C., Hughes, C., & West, D. (1988). Efficacy of cognitive behavior therapy and systematic desensitization in the treatment of rape trauma. *Behavior Therapy, 19,* 403–420.

Horowitz, M. (1976). *Stress response syndromes.* New York: Jason Aronson.

Kilpatrick, D. G., & Amick, A. E. (1985). Rape trauma. In M. Hersen & C. Last (Eds.), *Behavior therapy casebook* (pp. 86–103). New York: Springer.

Kilpatrick, D. G., Best, C. L., Veronen, J. L., Amick, A. E., Villeponteaux, L. A., & Ruff, G. A. (1985). Mental health correlates of criminal victimization: A random community survey. *Journal of Consulting and Clinical Psychology, 53,* 866–873.

Kilpatrick, D. G., Veronen, L. J., & Resick, P. A. (1982). Psychological sequelae to rape: Assessment and treatment strategies. In D. M. Doleys, R. L. Meredith, & A. R. Ciminero (Eds.), *Behavioral medicine: Assessment and treatment strategies* (pp. 473–498). New York: Plenum.

Koss, M. P., Gidycz, C. A., & Wisniewski, N. (1987). The scope of rape: Incidence and prevalence of sexual aggression and victimization in a national sample of higher education students. *Journal of Consulting and Clinical Psychology, 55,* 162–170.

Koss, M. P., & Harvey, M. (1991). *The rape victim: Clinical and community approaches to treatment* (2nd ed.). Lexington, MA: Stephen Greene Press.

McCann, I. L., & Pearlman, L. A. (1990). *Psychological trauma and the adult survivor: Theory, therapy and transformation.* New York: Brunner/Mazel.

Meichenbaum, D. H. (1985). *Stress inoculation training.* Elmsford, NY: Pergamon Press.

Resick, P. A., Jordan, C. G., Girelli, S. A., Hutter, C. K., & Marhoefer-Dvorak, S. (1988). A comparative outcome study of behavioral group therapy for sexual assault victims. *Behavior Therapy, 19,* 385-401.

Resick, P. A., Nishith, P., & Astin, M. (1996). Preliminary results of an outcome study comparing cognitive processing therapy and prolonged exposure. In P. Resick (Chair), *Treating sexual assault/sexual abuse pathology: Recent findings.* Symposium conducted at the annual convention of the Association for Advancement of Behavior Therapy, New York.

Resick, P. A., & Schnicke, M. K. (1990). Treating symptoms in adult survivors of sexual assault. *Journal of Interpersonal Violence, 5*(4), 488–506.

Resick, P. A., & Schnicke, M. K. (1992). Cognitive processing therapy for sexual assault victims. *Journal of Consulting and Clinical Psychology, 60,* 748–756.

Resick, P. A., & Schnicke, M. K. (1993). *Cognitive processing therapy for rape victims: A treatment manual.* Newbury Park, CA: Sage.

Roth, S., Dye, E., & Leibowitz, B. (1988). Group therapy for sexual assault victims. *Psychotherapy, 25,* 82–93.

Rothbaum, B. O., Foa, E. B., Riggs, D. S., Murdock, T., & Walsh, W. (1992). A prospective examination of post-traumatic stress disorder in rape victims. *Journal of Traumatic Stress, 3,* 455–475.

Chapter 4

Integrative Group Therapy With Disaster Workers

Raymond J. Emanuel and Robert J. Ursano

DISASTERS AND DISASTER WORKERS

The hallmark of all disasters is chaos. However, the human chaos of disasters is not random. Growing knowledge of individual, group, and community responses to disasters is leading to increased ability to describe, assess, and moderate disaster's impact on individuals and communities. Disaster workers include rescue workers and emergency medical personnel who are predictably exposed to disasters and their associated traumatic stressors in the line of duty (Ursano, Grieger, & McCarroll, 1996). The adverse effects of disaster cannot be judged solely on mortality rates or damage figures (Logue, 1996). Ultimately, the real toll is measured in terms of the physical and psychological disruption in every life that it affects.

The importance of this topic is underscored by the growing number of studies that have described crisis workers as at risk for numerous health problems associated with a wide variety of impairments in their occupational and social functioning. This group is unique in that some of their accepted day to day responsibilities place them in harm's way and expose them to potentially repetitive and cumulative trauma that may endanger their personal safety, health, and well being (Beaton, 1992).

Although the adverse effects of occupational exposure on disasters workers are recognized as constituting an important area of study, there is some disagreement within the disaster community regarding the extent of the problem. The majority of persons exposed to a disaster, victims and rescuers, alike, do well and have only mild, transitory symptoms. However, a minority of individuals do go on to develop behavioral and emotional symptoms or frank psychiatric illness post-disaster.

Recently, more attention has been focused on the lack of formalized preparation for dealing with the emotional responses that disaster workers encounter in the performance of those duties. The disaster workers themselves are aware that the potential adverse emotional impact on them is contingent on the type of event to which they are exposed (Hartsough & Myers, 1985). Unlike the victims of a disaster, disaster workers enter the disaster environment with a specific purpose and an ensemble of skills and logistic support to carry out their mission. They view themselves, not as victims helplessly subjected to overwhelming forces, but as rescuers. This identity as rescuers is nearly universal regardless of specific role, phase of entry into the relief work, or involvement with the victims (Flynn, 1996). The strong identity as rescuers contributes to both the resiliency and the vulnerability of disaster workers to post-traumatic stress.

This chapter will outline a theoretical framework that provides a basis for the practice of Integrative Group Treatment (IGT) with disaster workers and present examples of this concept in operational settings. The IGT framework views the individual as the transducer of environmental stressors contained within complex social systems prior to, during, and after a disaster. The interactions between the individual's unique physiology, his or her life experiences, the characteristics of these social networks, and the general and specific stressors to which he or she is exposed account for the syndromic nature of stress reactions and the wide variability in responses. This chapter will propose a theoretical model, IGT, in which the occupational stressors, individual differences, and multimodal interventions with disaster workers form a continuum of triage and treatment within the framework of the unique group dynamics of disaster workers.

TREATMENT ISSUES IN WORKING WITH DISASTER WORKERS

Effects of Stress on Individuals, Groups, and Organizations

Rituals of a professional group confer a powerful sense of group identity, group cohesion, and group norms. These rituals represent the mutual interdependence of the group members. Traumatic stress reactions, beyond their adverse effects on the individual, affect operational performance, i.e., group readiness and cohesion. Workers impaired by their response to stress are struggling not only with their psychological and somatic distress but also with their changing roles within the primary group as their occupational impairment results in their becoming more marginalized in the overall functioning of the organization (Orner, 1995).

Stress challenges the dynamic equilibrium of a system. Disasters stress homeostasis at every system level from the individual to the organizational and community levels. The fundamental goal of a group intervention is the restoration of homeostasis to the individual and throughout the social network.

At the individual level, the response to stress involves a complex, neuroendocrine stress response that is commonly known as the "fight or flight response." As much as two-thirds of the variance may be accounted for by genetic factors (Stratakis & Chrousos, 1995). Negative impact on an individual's sense of well being and performance or on both may occur when there is hypoarousal or hyperarousal of the stress response system (Chrousos & Gold, 1995). Individual genetic factors are only part of a complex system of stress adaptation. Multiple forces throughout the life span influence an individual's response at both the physiological and behavioral levels. Some of these other influences on stress response include: exposure to previous trauma (especially early in development); social learning; cognitive ability; interpersonal, occupational, and social skills; and the buffering effects of support systems.

The genetic diathesis of the individual and the characteristics of the event are etiologically important but are not amenable to therapeutic intervention. Aside from genetic and event-related variables, psychosocial deficits, cognitive appraisal, and social supports have a pronounced moderating effect on stress. Chrousos observed that, for social organisms, the development and maintenance of social bonds is critical to their survival and to the maintenance of homeostasis at all system levels (Chrousos & Gold, 1995). In light of this complex interaction between biology, event stressors, and psychosocial support systems, it is natural that psychosocial modalities, especially group interventions, have received increased attention as a method for ameliorating stress response at multiple levels.

Stressors Encountered by Disaster Workers

The therapist should have some field knowledge of the different types of stressors to which workers are routinely exposed and of their effects. Each category of stressor can have several components as summarized in Table 4.1.

The most fundamental type of stress to which disaster workers are exposed is physiological. Demands on disaster workers include long hours, irregular sleep cycles, poor access to potable water and food supplies, inadequate protection from the elements, and prolonged isolation from organizing information. Stress reactions can increase when there is an unfortunate confluence of adverse events, e.g., personal loss or injury, traumatic stimuli, and mission failure or human error.

Table 4.1. Stressors Experienced by Disaster Workers

Stressors	Characteristics	Responses or Effects
Physiological	Physical exertion, disrupted sleep, exposure to the elements, poor nutrition /hydration.	Exhaustion, increased dysfunction and job inefficiency, increased risk for injury.
Psychological	Actual or perceived risk of harm, contact with victims and survivors, exposure to the grotesque, isolation from social support.	Identification with victims, "Secondary Traumatic Stress," burn out, increased risk for persistent psychological and behavioral sequelae.
Occupational	Job-specific information overload, limits of ability "to rescue," apprehension about personal safety.	Feelings of inadequacy, anger, heroic efforts, minimization of dangerous job conditions, post-traumatic stress symptoms.
Organizational	Role conflict or ambiguity, Personal vs. Organizational needs, peer conflict, management labor issues.	Overall decrease in organizational effectiveness, increased hostility and frustration within and between organizational levels, erosion of group cohesion, loss of confidence in group support/isolation.

Psychological stress includes the risk, or presence of actual injury, and the persistent threat of harm, real and fantasized. In addition, psychological stress is increased by the extent of contact with the victims, the degree of success of rescue efforts (Genest, Levine, Ramsden, & Swanson, 1990), exposure to grotesque injury or remains, body handling, and the extent of contact with the survivors. (McCarroll, Ursano, Fullerton, & Lundy, 1995; McCarroll et al., 1993; Ursano et al., 1996; Ursano & McCarroll, 1990).

Effects on personal and professional functioning have been shown to present up to 18 months after a disaster (Weissberg & Katz, 1991). Every disaster challenges not only the individual disaster worker, but also, the organization itself. Organizations try to maintain an optimal flexibility to meet a wide range of disasters. However, they may still be overwhelmed with the unexpected intensity, speed, or scale of specific disasters. At times of maximal stress, individual and or organizational weaknesses may become magnified and interact in negative ways as outlined in Figure 4.1, which illustrates an Interactional Model of the Stressors and Stress Mediators.

MEDIATORS OF STRESS

Individual and Group Characteristics

There is conflicting evidence in literature regarding the contribution of personality characteristics and past experience to behavioral and psychological responses to disaster (see Table 4.2).

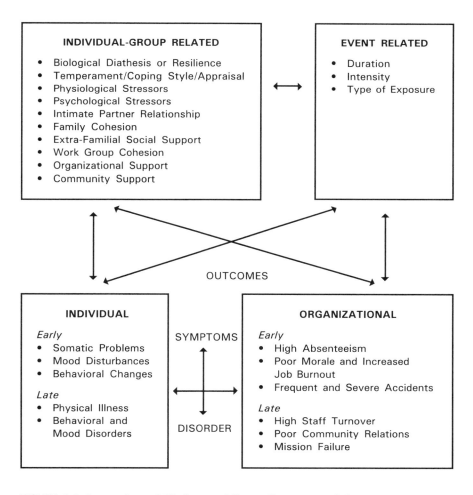

FIGURE 4.1. Interactions of Mediators of Stress Response and Outcomes

Table 4.2. Individual Mediating and Moderating Variables in Stress Response

	Risk of Maladaptive Response	Resiliency
Past Experiences	Curvilinear effect—risk increased at both ends of experience spectrum: increased if victim in the past; increased if history of intense reactions to past trauma.	Increased with moderate exposure/experience.
Chronic Stress levels present	Increased.	Decreased.
Personality Characteristics	Increased with immature defenses? Rigid Personality styles may be more at risk for being overwhelmed	Different personality types may offer protective effects
Stress Appraisal	Affected by level of training, temperament, sex, previous experience, life history, and current psychological state. In addition, factors such as educational level, social/cultural, coping style, and self-esteem of the individual influence appraisal.	

One point of view maintains that past experience may inoculate the worker against some of the adverse effects of exposure to traumatic events (Raphael, 1986), decrease anticipatory stress (McCarroll, 1995; McCarroll, 1993), or help to assimilate the event. It was observed in this group that firefighters with previous experience integrated the event better than the inexperienced firefighters (Hytten & Hasle, 1989). Weisaeth observed, following a paint factory fire, that those with previous experience in the merchant marines coped better and had less distress than those without previous exposure to disasters (Weisaeth, 1983).

Another viewpoint is that cumulative exposure may increase sensitization to traumatic stimuli and may be associated with a breakdown in coping (Mitchell, 1988; Moran & Britton, 1994). Beaton and Murphy's research with firefighters and paramedics failed to show any effect of past experience on any measure of stress (Beaton & Murphy, 1995). This suggests that the relationship between past experience and stress effects is curvilinear, with cumulative experience being protective up to a certain level of cumulative exposure after which it may contribute to sensitization and adverse effects.

It has also been shown that acute stress measures are influenced by chronic stress and that chronic stress explained 18% to 32% of the variance in psychological distress scales (Norris & Uhl, 1993). Further studies are needed to clarify the effects of repeated exposure to traumatic stress over a range of previous experiences and levels of exposures.

Most studies of disaster workers have found a relationship between disaster work and psychiatric symptoms. Despite increasing interest, little is known about the contribution of individual personality differences. It does not appear that emergency workers have hardier personality characteristics when compared to nonemergency worker normals (Moran & Britton, 1994). Current symptomatology in emergency workers was most strongly associated with the frequency of past incidents as a victim, immature defensive style, and the intensity of reaction to past traumatic incident (Moran & Britton, 1994).

Beyond the physical and intellectual demands imposed by the occupational tasks, a disaster takes on a specific meaning to the individual. This process by which disasters take on particular meaning is influenced by an individual's temperament, sex, previous experience, life history, and current psychological state. In addition, factors such as educational level, social and cultural, coping style, and self-esteem may contribute to an individual's vulnerability or resiliency (McCarroll et al., 1995; McFarlane, 1986).

Occupational Characteristics

Disaster workers may also experience role conflict when their personal needs or reactions conflict with the demands of the organizational task. Personal reactions to suffering or irate victims may contradict expected responses in those situations. Different ideas about the how a job should be performed can lead to conflict between colleagues and between supervisors and workers. The heightened emotions and extraordinary demands resulting from a disaster may increase feelings of role confusion and task some individuals with responsibilities outside their usual area of expertise (Hartsough & Myers, 1985).

Social Mediators

Social supports are important moderating factors after a disaster. Single parents may be at a higher risk for developing psychiatric disorders, since they often have fewer resources to begin with and loose some after a disaster (Solomon, Smith, Robins, & Fischbach, 1987). Limited support resources with persistent financial hardship and limited employment opportunities may lead to increase in family violence, spouse abuse, and child abuse with high morbidity and significant mortality (Solomon et al., 1987).

Event Characteristics

Perhaps the best predictor of the probability and the frequency of psychiatric illness is the severity of the traumatic event (Ursano, 1996; Pynoos, 1993). Psychiatric morbidity has also been documented in association with exposure to the injured and dying (Beaton & Murphy, 1995; Ursano, Fullerton, & Kao, 1995a).

WHY DO INTEGRATIVE GROUP TREATMENT?

Treatment Goals

IGT is directed towards decreasing pain and suffering, optimizing performance and recovery, and it is hoped, decreasing the possibility of developing chronic dysfunction. Emergency worker groups and their families are subject to multiple consequences after a disaster. Disaster workers are also at increased risk for physical illness, social impairment, and performance breakdown. Clinical characterization of the severity and chronicity of the symptoms is important but may be complicated by persistent minimization of symptoms early in the course of the disorder and by the delayed onset of symptomatology that is commonly observed.

The effects of the initial emotional reactions to a dramatic event may not be pronounced for the individual or the organization. Some early reactions include anxiety, fear, anger, irritability, hopelessness, and melancholy. For most people, these initial symptoms resolve with time. For others, however, these symptoms diminish but may evolve into chronic, smoldering, emotional distress or a clearly identifiable psychiatric disorder. The psychic numbing and withdrawal seen in some rescue workers can impair their ability to maintain their normal social relationships, further depriving them of support when they may most need it and impairing recovery and the ability to return to work.

PTSD is estimated to develop in 10% to 30% of highly exposed individuals, and it can have dire human and financial costs to individuals and organizations. Although PTSD receives much of the attention in trauma research, as the National Comorbidity Study has shown, comorbidity is the rule rather than the exception. Epstein has suggested that the avoidant symptoms of PTSD may delay or preclude the diagnosis of the disorder unless frequent follow-ups are performed after the trauma (Epstein, 1993). Major depression, generalized anxiety disorder, and adjustment disorders are less studied but probably occur at higher rates in the aftermath of a disaster than has been appreciated (Rundell, Ursano, Holloway, & Silberman, 1989). Substance abuse is frequently comorbid with other psychiatric illnesses and, given the possible increased use in disaster workers (Hartsough & Myers, 1985) is a potential chronic outcome.

Intra- or Interorganizational conflict can also result after a disaster and such conflict can decrease the overall efficiency of the organizational effort. It places the individual worker under greater stress, often further reducing the overall functioning of the organization.

This impairment of the organization can manifest itself in low morale, high absenteeism, job burnout, and substandard performance, which if allowed to persist may evolve into increased severity or frequency of job-related accidents or frequent mission failures. For all these reasons, an integrative group treatment approach that links primary to secondary and tertiary interventions is indicated as part of a disaster response.

Cost Benefit Analysis

In an era intensely concerned with cost containment and measurable treatment outcomes, the first questions that might be raised about group interventions for disaster workers might be: How much will it cost? How will it benefit us? Will it achieve results? All three of these questions pose difficulties in giving definitive answers. However, it is becoming clearer that there are significant costs of not attending to the adverse effects of traumatic exposure on emergency workers. This cost can be measured in the loss of emergency workers to serious emotional and physical disorders, dysfunctional interpersonal relationships, substance abuse, and shortened careers. In addition, the causes of 75% to 85% of all industrial accidents are related to fatigue, poor concentration, and inattentiveness (Jones & Dubois, 1987). These work-related accidents in the U.S.A. had an estimated cost of $32 billion dollars in 1982. Psychological and psychosomatic problems contribute to over 60% of long-term employee disability cases and approximately 11% of all occupational disease claims are for workplace stress (Jones & Dubois, 1987). The routine exposure to psychological and physical stressors places the disaster worker in a very high risk category.

INTEGRATIVE GROUP TREATMENT (IGT)

Definition

Integrative Group Treatment for disaster workers is based on the principles of preventive medicine. IGT is not one specific treatment but rather a spectrum of interdependent group interventions, extending from primary prevention strategies to tertiary group treatment. The strategies include organizational and community consultation and outreach programs with the goals of identifying high-risk groups, promoting individual and group recovery, and minimizing performance breakdown and group disruption (Ursano, Fullerton, & Norwood, 1995b).

The full spectrum of IGT interventions is shown in Figure 4.2. The general concept of IGT is that the success of any intervention is linked to a comprehensive program of group interventions that becomes incorporated into the organizational work culture. This approach gives the program design flexibility, basing itself on the needs and resources of the organization while providing a basic conceptual foundation. IGT maximizes clinical and cost effective treatment by beginning with a thorough assessment and focused treatment interventions.

IGT begins with consideration of primary IGT modalities prior to any disaster. In this phase, primary prevention is emphasized. Almost all primary interventions commonly used in stress prevention or reduction among disaster workers are intrinsically group processes that involve many, if not all, of the members of the organization who are at risk. The wide range of these activities include: training and education, after-action debriefings, and family and community support.

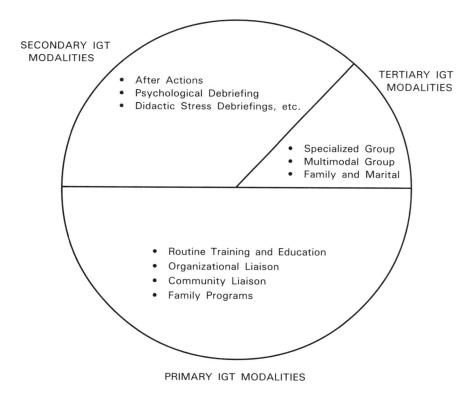

Figure 4.2. Integrative Group Treatment Modalities

IGT secondary modalities are utilized after the event. There are three central considerations in the assessment and treatment plan formulation at this stage: (a) risk estimate associated with the severity of the trauma exposure, (b) identifications of individuals at risk, and (c) identification of available social support resources. If the event is of routine intensity and duration, routine debriefing techniques and informal social support may be all that is required.

Shalev (1995) has outlined several types of debriefing. Task-oriented debriefings are commonly used in large organizations and are not necessarily related to trauma exposure. They serve the purpose of pooling information or lessons learned from a particular event. This type of established activity in an organization can serve as a nice link to a traumatic debriefing should one become necessary in the organization (Shalev, 1995).

For events that are of greater severity, are marked by unusual loss or threat, or involve high-risk individuals, more formal IGT debriefing techniques may be indicated. The techniques of psychological group debriefing are most often connected with the work of B. Raphael and J. Mitchell. Psychological debriefings and Critical Incident Stress Debriefing (CISD) are similarly based on the hypothesis that the event's cognitive structure is modified through retelling and by experiencing an emotional release, thereby preventing or reducing the risk of more serious stress reactions. Other hoped for beneficial effects include enhancing group cohesion and the general mobilization of social support (Shalev, 1995).

Variations in the format of debriefings, differences in organizational culture, varying symptomatology of the subjects, psychiatric comorbidity, and multiple types of stress exposure, have made evaluation of the effectiveness of these interventions challenging. The most detailed follow-up study to date is Kenardy et al. (1996). This study demonstrated that those who were not debriefed showed a more rapid reduction of their General Health Questionnaire scores over time. Examination of the characteristics of the subjects in this study suggest that personality, sensitivity and neuroticism may increase reactivity following the trauma with debriefing.

IGT secondary modalities require consideration of the role of families and spouses in initiating, facilitating, and maintaining recovery from stress. The impact of the trauma on the family of a disaster worker can be the virtual loss of that individual as a spouse or parent or both. This loss of an integral member of the family can then become part of a vicious cycle in which there is a collapse of the recovery environment further exacerbating the dysfunction of the individual and the family. Family therapy and possibly adjunctive marital therapy should be a consideration in some cases in order to restore the recovery environment of the disaster worker.

Family education about the emotional and behavioral impact of disaster work on workers can be used to maintain strong social support systems. Fullerton and Ursano (1996) have shown that caretaking of disaster workers by spouses is common and stressful. Disaster worker's wives have higher levels of intrusive and avoidant symptoms (Ursano et al., 1996). By providing support to spouses and altering the recovery environments one hopes to reduce the risk of the development of chronic symptomatology. In general, it is important to note that marital happiness has been observed to contribute far more toward global happiness than any other variable, and friends and family are generally seen as more trusted than professionals (Colins & Pancoast, 1976). Thus, enhancement and use of naturally occurring social supports after a disaster is expected to be associated with lower levels of psychopathology (Ursano et al., 1996).

IGT also includes recognition of risks in post-disaster interactions. Socially mediated responses to disaster may have both negative and positive aspects. Solomon et al. (1987) studied individuals either personally or indirectly exposed to disaster and found that males and females differed in their response to disaster exposure. Victims who were both personally exposed to disaster and heavily relied upon by their social network were far more likely to somatizise (females) or abuse alcohol (males) than personally exposed individuals with more moderate network demands. Spouse support moderated male symptomatology but exacerbated symptoms of female victims. The result suggested that, particularly in women, the negative consequences of strong social ties can outweigh the supportive effects in times of extreme stress (Solomon et al., 1987).

IGT tertiary group modalities are defined as therapy for small groups of individuals (4-8 members) who have been identified as having persistent mood and behavioral symptoms associated with exposure to a traumatic occupational event. At the tertiary level, these groups utilize many of the psychodynamic processes operating in primary and secondary groups but with increased intensity and focus. The smaller process-oriented group can promote more intimate sharing and allow for more individualized support. However, because of the increased intensity of this process, individuals who are marginally coping with their affect may not be candidates for this type of group but may require other more specialized treatments (e.g., individual psychotherapy or pharmacotherapy or both).

Outcome studies of tertiary group psychotherapy techniques for individuals exposed to traumatic stressors have generally focused on PTSD related to combat, and, even then, they are meager (Solomon, Gerrity, & Muff, 1992a). The range of tertiary groups addressing PTSD include: process groups, cognitive-behavioral, psychoeducational, psychoanalytical, Jungian dream work, and psychodrama (Allen & Bloom, 1994). Most inpatient treatment programs have been done with combat veterans and are multimodal therapies (Solomon et al., 1992a; Solomon, Bleich, Shoham, Nardi, & Kotler, 1992b).

A study of the incorporation of psychological debriefing techniques within a brief group psychotherapy program by Busuttil et al. (1995) found that 29 out of 34 subjects who were initially positive for PTSD no longer met DSM-III-R criteria at one year follow-up. Notably, as with most of the studies in this area, this was an open outcome study. This study also incorporated the use of medications and family or marital therapy. This study's four main strategies were: (a) a comprehensive assessment, (b) a structured group therapy format, (c) Medications prescribed as indicated, and (d) long-term follow-up reviews at six-week, six-month and one-year intervals. This program was relatively labor intensive. The formal group work included two primary therapists and a support therapist and spanned 63 hours.

This study exemplifies some of the methodological difficulties in trying to ascertain the efficacy of "pure" group therapy. The average duration of PTSD in this study was two years (range from one month to 31 years). No details regarding previous treatment trials were given for any of the subjects. All eight subjects (about one quarter of all subjects) who received medication were started on medications during the study's follow-up period. Comorbid psychopathology was evaluated by self-report questionnaires. The observation that none of the subjects reported the use of illicit drugs and there was no significant change in alcohol consumption in any of the assessment intervals may indicate that this was a relatively psychologically healthy group of individuals with PTSD symptomatology, i.e., without some of the serious comorbidity, particularly substance abuse, that is often associated with PTSD.

As the intensity of treatment increases, as with tertiary group intervention, so does the labor intensity and cost. Because of the present lack of empirical studies both caution and clinical wisdom are needed in applying debriefing and multimodal techniques. It is generally appreciated that some individuals will require specialized individual therapy for treatment of substance dependence, or major affective, anxiety, and personality disorders, or combinations of these.

IGT: AN EXAMPLE OF AN IGT SECONDARY INTERVENTION

The following example describes an IGT intervention. In July, 1996, TWA Flight 800, carrying 212 passengers and 17 crew members, exploded and crashed into the Atlantic Ocean off the coast of Long Island shortly after taking off from New York City's John F. Kennedy International Airport en route to Paris. There were no survivors, and, at this time, the cause of the crash has not been determined. Military and civilian divers from the region were enlisted in the efforts to recover the remains of the victims and to salvage the plane wreckage.

The consulting organization had a program that provided access to a disaster support team at all times. The line supervisor for one of these teams of divers requested this service for two groups of divers that had worked at the crash site on two separate occasions. He was supported by upper management to obtain this service through consultation procedures already existing within the organization. Premeeting discussion about the stressors to which the men had been exposed and whether or not there were any particular concerns revealed that the first group of divers (about 12 men) had worked long hours under adverse weather and working conditions, that they had experienced their working environment as unsafe, and that they thought the head of their operation lacked knowledge of their specialty. The stated reason for the debriefing was the hope of preventing any adverse sequelae to the divers rather than to address any specific problem that was apparent at the time.

Within one week after the men finished their salvage work, two consultants met with each group of divers for about two hours in the conference room of the main dive facility located about 200 miles from the crash site. The men were all experienced divers and ranged in age from late 20s to early 40s. In establishing the focus as a secondary group intervention—working with individuals at risk but without identified illness or dysfunction—it was explained to them that the group leaders were not experts in diving, nor were we there as mental health providers or as fact finders for the organization. We told them that we were there simply to listen to their dive experiences at the crash site and to whatever associated thoughts, feelings, or questions they had regarding the experience, and that anonymity would be maintained.

The group's initial reaction was one of apprehension mixed with distrust. None of the men had been through anything more than routine operational debriefing before, and they all had some reservations about the purpose or need for the two nondiver leaders to know about their experiences on this dive. It was extremely important that the lead supervisor, with whom the group had a trusting relationship, reiterated his support for the session and even led off with some of his impressions and feelings about the operation. This greatly facilitated others in expressing their opinions.

The first statements about the experience generally reflected attempts to minimize the stressors and minimized any traumatic exposure as "part of the job." Then the descriptions became more focused on the particulars of this disaster, first in terms of the general working conditions and safety issues, and then in terms of the more traumatic aspects of personal exposure. For many, the personalization of the exposure led to associations with previous experiences. With the retelling of experiences from previous dives, there were simultaneously renewed efforts to minimize the current experience at the same time strong affects associated with previous experiences were being expressed. Each experience related by individual members also appeared to strengthen the bond between them as professionals and as a particular group of divers.

The experience of being safe during the personal disclosure of professional experiences allowed for a gradual sharing of more personal feelings related to these experiences and a recognition that intense feelings—not their absence—were part of the "normal" response. One diver related how he had been unable to eat crabs since seeing them totally scavenge the flesh off victims' bones on the ocean floor. Another related that finding personal effects of the victims like wallets with photographs was more traumatic than dealing with the dead bodies of victims. One diver recalled his feelings of sadness when a man, who had lost his wife and two children, held up a sign thanking the divers for their efforts.

The expression of this emotion was often accompanied spontaneously by disclosures that the person usually relied on talking with his spouse or friends in order to deal with his feelings. Other divers readily admitted that they did not feel comfortable talking to anyone about their experiences. For these divers, their outlet was in their recreation away from work. One individual who had not spoken throughout the session voiced his complaint that there was not a debriefing at the dive site. The general group reaction was negative to his comment and some tension developed within the group. The tension was never totally resolved within the session. Afterwards, the supervisor related that this individual had had some alcohol-related problems at work. An offer was made to meet with the individual privately if he desired. The group ended by reasserting the normalcy of the experience. However, included in this normalization of the experience was a clear recognition of the effects, an appreciation for the experience of the group and support available both within and outside the group and organization.

ANALYSIS OF THE IGT INTERVENTION

IGT Primary Modalities: Organizational Preparation and Liaison

The success of small group interventions is directly related to the successful liaison work with the leaders of the organization. This preparatory work helps define the hurdles that behavioral health workers need to overcome before any effective interventions can be undertaken. The first is a near universal fear of stigmatization or being labeled as "weak" or "crazy" if you require mental health services. This is heightened by an occupational environment that imposes high standards and expectations of self-reliance to overcome emotional distress. Also, there is the understandable concern about confidentiality and possible ramifications on career opportunities. In the above example, the most important work had been done prior to the intervention. The organization had removed some of the initial obstacles through education of its supervisory personnel, incorporation of the debriefing procedure within routine operations, and ready access of an intervention team. Still the natural reluctance to opening up to outsiders and questions of confidentially had to be addressed. Managers of disaster relief are often supportive of the stress management efforts but may see the support as for their workers and not applicable to themselves. The direct supportive involvement of management in this group greatly increased the chances for a successful intervention.

Usually, the preparation of the individual members is done through the organization. In this case, this preparation was accomplished through a predisaster commitment by the organization to educate their workers about the importance and possible need for a variety of efforts to prevent the adverse consequences of stress exposure. However, this ideal situation is rarely obtained. The vignette is an example of an organization that had, as part of its overall disaster response plan interventions for its exposed workers, a protocol that essentially presented all those exposed to the disaster site for a preliminary debriefing. Although there was some initial confusion about how to access the support from middle management, strong encouragement and direction from upper level management were provided. As opposed to individual interviews of potential group members, the members of the divers group were essentially told to attend a debriefing. Their knowledge of what this might entail was nominal. This points out that even in preplanned and organizationally-supported programs, front line workers may still have little understanding of the role of debriefing,

IGT Secondary Modalities: Small Group Interventions

Group Selection   Group dynamics among disaster workers are quite complex. Disaster worker personnel frequently change, requiring individuals to work through feelings of unfamiliarity and competition in order to establish a trusting working relationship within a short time period. But even this group identity, forged by the intensity and necessities of disaster work, is soon broken up by the endless series of goodbyes that accompanies disaster work. An ever-changing work group composition can sometimes result in the ambiguous roles and the tension that poorly defined boundaries can bring to individuals and groups. Alternatively, change may occasionally limit the extent of dysfunctional interpersonal interactions.

In this group of divers, the men had worked as a team on other occasions and were expecting to participate together in the future. With an intimate ongoing team like this one, the de facto functioning group brings both the advantages and disadvantages of preexisting relationships among the group members. The nature of the occupational settings and characteristics of this group usually make traditional long-term group therapy impractical if not impossible within the organizational setting. For this reason, IGT emphasizes the interdependence and continuity of group work at different intervention levels.

A homogeneous group of disaster workers, who have all been exposed to similar traumatic stimuli in the line of duty, offers the benefit of peer support and inherent group cohesion. Schachter (1959) observed that his subjects preferred to share the company of persons facing the same stressful situation. This support process is thought to develop because peers have the opportunity to share their stressful experiences. It highlights the stress moderating impact of empathy, normalization, and validation (Gottlieb, 1996; Schachter, 1959). Emotional ventilation has been shown to mitigate feelings of deviance and depression, producing a normalizing effect that would not likely have occurred through interactions with individuals who had not been subjected to the same stressful encounter (Coates & Winston, 1983; Gottlieb, 1996). A disadvantage of a homogeneous group from the same profession is that the group expectations may inhibit an individual from expressing certain thoughts, feelings, or vulnerabilities that are incongruent with the prevailing professional culture. However, the therapist can attempt to counter this tendency by helping the group to verbalize in a general abstract way what the group taboos are.

Heterogeneous groups may have the advantage of reducing feelings of uniqueness, isolation, and social withdrawal (Scaturo & Hardoby, 1988). A heterogeneous group, with members from outside the disaster worker's community or composed of nontraumatized members, may be able to draw the traumatized individual's focus out beyond the traumatic experience. In this way, the disaster worker may more easily ameliorate his or her traumatic experience by reexperiencing the positive, life-affirming aspects of his or her life.

Many of the members of the divers group considered the commander of the operation to be inexperienced in their area and to be unnecessarily exposing them to high levels of risk. In this group, middle management was represented by an on-site supervisor. This individual had the uncomfortable position of identification with both the issues of the front line workers and those of upper management. However, he could help the group by serving as a bridge between those different viewpoints.

Treatment Phases

Opening Phase   The initial phases of both debriefing and intensive group work are similar in that the establishment of a safe environment and trust in the therapist are key components. The group will try to define more clearly the role and expertise of the therapist if that is not already clearly established and accepted.

As is commonly the case, in this example, issues related to confidentiality were integral in establishing a safe group environment. In working with disaster workers, the group therapist needs to consider issues beyond the normal rules of confidentiality. Even if confidentiality is maintained, information disclosed in the group can have unforeseen impact. The interpersonal relationships among disaster workers, especially from the same organization, are both personal and professional. The therapist may have to monitor more tightly what degree of personal disclosure is safe in this setting. There is a fine line between knowing enough about an individual to have confidence in him or her and having too much personal information that may interfere with an ongoing professional relationship. Personal disclosure may be more likely and more appropriate in groups in which there is a sense of ultimate termination and geographic separation of the group members. However, the therapist must consider that the mobility and fluidity of the disaster worker community, as in this group, makes recontact in another working relationship between members of the group very likely.

Who sponsors the therapeutic work often raises issues of confidentiality. In this example, it was the work group supervisor. This relationship may define the tone and atmosphere in which the group work proceeds. Is the group sponsored by the local organization of the disaster workers or "the main office"? Sponsorship may or may not be equivalent to organizational support for disaster workers to seek treatment. Administrators may feel pressured by the political correctness not to object to treatment for disaster workers, but they may indirectly or passively discourage participation. Who the therapist works for may affect to what extent the therapist is viewed as a group member or an outsider; and it may also reflect his or her own biases. Perception of the therapist as a member of the disaster worker community may help establish trust and credibility but may further inhibit disclosure of information repressed generally by the organizational culture.

Middle Phase   To paraphrase Freud, in therapy, like chess, only the opening and closing moves allow for a systematic presentation. In the middle, there is the infinite variety of permutations. In this case, the focus on the management or mismanagement of the salvage operation was an important bridge to feelings of fear, anger, and helplessness among the divers. As the discussion proceeded, the focus shifted from safety issues, which were eventually recognized by the group as not significantly different from previous operations, to the issues of anticipatory anxiety, guilt from the "enjoyment" of the work, anger over breakup of unit cohesiveness and unnecessarily long hours.

Eventually, the divers were able to discuss how exposure to the personal effects of the victims or even the communication of gratitude from relatives of the victims evoked feelings related to the divers own families, their previous dives, and the subtle ways that the experience had, at least transiently, changed their lives. Likewise, individual members of any group may be more comfortable initiating the discussion of their feelings with issues that have group recognition and approval and that are relatively safe. The therapist tries to ensure that the group will not remain fixated at this stage of the group process. As the group progresses, the working with more personal issues that is done by some individuals provides a model and gives permission for the more reticent members to discuss their own personal reactions. As is usually the case, the facilitating efforts of the therapist must be balanced by respect for the readiness of individuals to disclose their feelings. Debriefers and group leaders should recognize that reticence may be an appropriate defense for an individual who is not yet ready for this type of disclosure; but it may also be a sign of an increasing isolation from the group. Caplan has remarked that the "native patterns and timetables" of the adjustment process in each individual must be respected and preconceived notions about what constitutes "normal" reactions or grieving process should not be too rigid (Caplan, 1976). Group leaders may primarily facilitate the optimum sharing of experience in the group by maintaining an atmosphere of safety and support. The mutual aid that was experienced in this group allowed the members of the group to alternate between the roles of helper and help recipient by validating each others' experiences and enhancing their own esteem as well as that of others. Even the simple expression of emotion in this group appeared to confirm Pennebaker's (1984) observation about the positive impact of emotional ventilation on mood states. At the level of cognitive restructuring, this group was able to reframe their exposure to the dangerousness of the work and the tragedies of the families of the victims within the broader context of their own lives and work. Janoff-Bulman's found that support groups like this one can assist individuals to reestablish meaning when life crises have shattered their assumptions about the world (Gottlieb, 1996; Janoff-Bulman, 1992; Pennebaker & O'Heeron, 1984; Silver & Wortman, 1980).

Termination   Termination brings members of the group back to a normalization of their experience based on an integration of individual, group, and organizational perspectives (rather than denial and misinformation). At termination, the internalization of the shared group experience of the traumatic exposure is reinforced. This shared group experience ameliorates the isolating effects of traumatic exposure by confirmation of the survivability of disaster workers and placing the trauma in the context of the larger experience of the group.

IGT CONTINUITY: ONGOING TRIAGE AND TREATMENT

It is important to recall that before, during, and after secondary or tertiary IGT interventions, regular monitoring of individual and organizational functioning is needed. This monitoring provides a barometer of health for the individual and the group. Dysfunction can serve as an early warning that increases in education, support, or specialized treatment may be needed. The individual in this example who was having work and possible alcohol abuse problems typifies this type of triage at a secondary IGT group intervention level.

CONCLUSION

The social and interpersonal nature of groups provides an ideal environment for the repair of "schemas for safety, trust, dependency, independence, power, self-esteem, and intimacy" (Allen & Bloom, 1994). IGT work with disaster workers includes all of the challenges common to devising and studying mental health interventions for the large number of people exposed to traumatic events. Disaster workers are not the typical self-referred client or patient population. Their event stressors are often more public, at times even national news. The stressor is usually beyond that experienced by the average person. The stress of this exposure is not only filtered through the unique characteristics of the individual but also through the dominant culture and conventions of the group to which he or she belongs.

At a societal level, individuals in the emergency and rescue profession share some powerful myths: "Heroes do not or should not have any problems," and "Time heals all wounds" (Scurfield, 1992). These cultural beliefs are a prominent part of the disaster worker community and can delay or preclude the identification of psychiatric problems.

Disaster workers are at increased risk for post-traumatic stress reactions because of the nature of their occupational exposure. The routine occupational stress of disaster workers can be placed on the continuum of job stress that even in its more mundane forms has been associated with significant individual and organizational morbidity. Most individuals, including disaster workers, exposed to trauma have transient stress reactions with uneventful recoveries. Some individuals, however, develop chronic symptoms and meet the criteria for one or more psychiatric disorders.

IGT is not a single intervention but a spectrum of strategies based on the principles of group and organizational dynamics within the context of the unique characteristics of disaster workers and their organizations. IGT begins preexposure with interventions for large groups of asymptomatic individuals. IGT then extends to specialized treatments initiated post-disaster, focusing on small groups of symptomatic individuals. At all levels, IGT uses assessment strategies to guide the judicious use of interventions. Preexposure, IGT primary intervention requires that the organization develop training and screening programs to identify those individuals who are at increased risk by history or behavioral characteristics and implement programs designed to reduce those risks. These programs promote a healthy lifestyle, stress management, and rigorous skills training. IGT primary interventions form the foundation on which interventions with the disaster community must rest.

Post-exposure, IGT secondary modalities include the various types of debriefings and after actions. Tertiary IGT group modalities are the specialized treatment of individuals triaged during the process of a secondary IGT interventions. IGT tertiary interventions can be customized to the organizational and situational needs and resource constraints of the organization. This level of group intervention is indicated for those individuals whose social and occupational dysfunction persist.

Because of the occupational risks to disaster workers for serious adverse outcome to intense and chronic exposure or both, to traumatic events, a wide variety of interventions are used with increasing frequency. Currently, there is little clear outcome data for support of the multifaceted IGT components. The importance of the IGT approach is that it provides a conceptual integration that has not been previously present. The challenge of the future is to provide an empirical base for this theoretical framework that can further guide the design, coordination, and implementation of interventions and also be understandable and practical to the individuals and organizations served.

REFERENCES

Allen, S. N., & Bloom, S. L. (1994). Group and family treatment of post-traumatic stress disorder. *Psychiatric Clinics of North America, 17*(2), 425–437.

Beaton, R., & Murphy, S. (1995). Working with people in crisis: Research implications. In C. Figley (Ed.), *Compassion fatigue: Coping with secondary traumatic stress disorder in those who treat the traumatized* (Vol. 1, pp. 51–81). New York: Brunner/Mazel.

Birk, L. (1974). Intensive group therapy: An effective behavioral-pyschoanalytical method. *American Journal of Pyschiatry, 131,* 11–16.

Busuttil, W., Turnbull, G. J., Neal, L. A., Rollins, J., West, A. G., Blanch, N., & Herepath, R. (1995). Incorporating psychological debriefing techniques within a brief group psychotherapy programme for the treatment of post-traumatic stress disorder. *British Journal of Psychiatry, 167,* 495–502.

Caplan, G. (1976). Organization of support systems for civilian populations. In G. Kaplan & M. Killilea (Eds.), *Support systems and mutual help* (pp. 273–315). New York: Grune & Stratton.

Chrousos, G. P., & Gold, P. W. (1995). Introduction (Vol. 771). New York: New York Academy of Sciences.

Coates, D., & Winston, T. (1983). Counteracting the deviance of depression: Peer support groups for victims. *Journal of Social Issues, 39,* 169.

Colins, A. G., & Pancoast, D. L. (1976). *Natural helping networks: A strategy for prevention.* Washington DC: National Association of Social Workers.

Epstein, R. S. (1993). Avoidant symptoms cloaking the diagnosis of PTSD in patients with severe accidental injury. *Journal of Traumatic Stress, 6*(4), 451–458.

Flynn, B. (1996). Chief emergency services and disaster relief branch. Personal communication.

Genest, M., Levine, J., Ramsden, V., & Swanson, R. (1990). The impact of providing help: Emergency workers and cardiopulmonary resuscitation attempts. *Journal of Traumatic Stress, 3*(2), 305–313.

Gottlieb, B. H. (1996). Theories and practices of mobilizing support in stressful circumstances. In C. L. Cooper (Ed.), *Stress, medicine, and health* (Vol. 1, pp. 339–374). Boca Raton, FL: CRC Press.

Hartsough, D., & Myers, D. G. (1985). *Disaster work and mental health: Prevention and control of stress among workers.* Rockville, MD: National Institute of Mental Health.

Hytten, K., & Hasle, A. (1989). Firefighters: A study of stress and coping. *Actapsychiatr. scand, Supplement 355*(80), 50–55.

Janoff-Bulman, R. (1992). *Shattered assumptions.* New York: The Free Press.

Jones, J. W., & Dubois, D. (1987). A review of organizational stress assessment instruments. In L. R. Murphy & T. F. Schoenborn (Eds.), *Stress management in work settings* (pp. 47–66). Washington, DC: U.S. Department of Health and Human Services.

Kenardy, J. A., Webster, R. A., Lewin, T. J., Carr, V. J., Hazell, P. L., & Carter, G. L. (1996). Stress debriefing and patterns of recovery following a natural disaster. *Journal of Traumatic Stress, 9*(1), 37–49.

Logue, J. N. (1996). Disasters, the environment, and public health: Improving our response. *American Journal of Public Health, 86*(9), 1207–1210.

McCarroll, J., Ursano, R., Fullerton, C., & Lundy, A. (1995). Anticipatory stress of handling human remains from the Persian Gulf War. *The Journal of Nervous and Mental Disease, 183*(11), 700–705.

McCarroll, J., Ursano, R., Ventis, W., Fullerton, C., Oates, G., Friedman, H., Shean, G., & Wright, K. (1993). Anticipation of handling the dead: Effects of gender and experience. *British Journal of Psychology, 32,* 466–468.

McFarlane, A. C. (1986). The longitudinal course of post-traumatic morbidity: The range of outcomes and their predictors. *Journal of Nervous and Mental Disease, 176,* 30–39.

Mitchell, J. (1988). The impact of stress on emergency service personnel: Policy issues in emergency response. In L. Comfort (Ed.), *Managing disasters: Strategies and policy perspectives.*

Moran, C., & Britton, N. (1994). Emergency work experience and reactions to traumatic incidents. *Journal of Traumatic Stress, 7*(4), 575–585.

Norris, F. H., & Uhl, G. A. (1993). Chronic stress as a mediator of acute stress: The case of Hurricane Hugo. *Journal of Applied Social Psychology, 23*(16), 1263–1284.

Orner, R. J. (1995). Intervention strategies for emergency response groups: A new conceptual framework. In S. E. Hobfol & M. W. de Vries (Eds.), *Extreme stress and communities: Impact and intervention.* Dordrecht: Kluwer Academic Publishers.

Pennebaker, J. W., & O'Heeron, R. C. (1984). Confiding in others and illness rate among spouses of suicide and accidental death victims. *Journal of Abnormal Psychology, 93*(473).

Raphael, B. (1986). *When disaster strikes: A handbook for caring professions.* London: Hutchinson.

Rundell, J. R., Ursano, R. J., Holloway, H. C., & Silberman, E. K. (1989). Psychiatric response to trauma. *Hospital and Community Psychiatry, 401*(1), 68–74.

Scaturo, D. J., & Hardoby, W. J. (1988). Psychotherapy with traumatized Vietnam combatants: an overview of individual, group, and family treatment modalities. *Military Medicine, 153,* 262–269.

Schachter, S. (1959). *The psychology of affiliation.* Palo Alto, CA: Stanford University Press.

Scurfield, R. M. (1992). The collusion of sanitization and silence about war: An aftermath of "Operation Desert Storm." *Journal of Traumatic Stress, 5*(3), 505–512.

Shalev, A. (1995). Debriefing following traumatic exposure. In R. J. Ursano, C. S. Fullerton, & B. G. McCaughey (Eds.), *Individual and community responses to trauma and disaster: The structure of human chaos* (2nd ed., Vol. 1, pp. 3–27). London: Cambridge University Press.

Silver, R. L., & Wortman, C. B. (1980). Copying with undesirable life events. In J. Garber & M. E. Seligman (Eds.), *Human helplessness: Theory and applications* (p. 279). New York: Academic Press.

Solomon, S. D., Gerrity, E. T., & Muff, A. A. (1992a). Efficacy of treatments for post-traumatic stress disorder. *Journal of the American Medical Association, 268,* 633–638.

Solomon, S. D., Smith, E. M., Robins, L. N., & Fischbach, R. L. (1987). Social involvement as a mediator of disaster-induced stress. *Journal of Applied Social Psychology, 17*(12), 1092–1112.

Solomon, Z., Bleich, A., Shoham, S., Nardi, C., & Kotler, M. (1992b). The "Koach" project for treatment of combat-related PTSD: Aims and methodology. *Journal of Traumatic Stress, 5*(2), 175–193.

Stratakis, C. A., & Chrousos, G. P. (1995). *Neuroendocrinology of the stress system* (Vol. 771). New York: New York Academy of Sciences.

Ursano, R., Fullerton, C., & Kao, T. C. (1995a). Longitudinal assessment of post-traumatic stress disorder and depression after exposure to traumatic death. *The Journal of Nervous and Mental Disease, 42,* 36–42.

Ursano, R., Fullerton, C., & Norwood, A. (1995b). Psychiatric dimensions of disaster: Patient care, community consultation, and preventive medicine. *Harvard Review of Psychiatry, 39*(1), 196–209.

Ursano, R., Grieger, T., & McCarroll, E. (1996). Prevention of post traumatic stress: Consultation, training, and early treatment. In B.A. van der Kolk, A.C. McFarlane, & L. Weisaeth (Eds.), *Traumatic stress: The effects of overwhelming experience on mind, body, and society* (pp. 411–462). New York: The Guilford Press.

Ursano, R., & McCarroll, J. (1990). The nature of traumatic stressors: Handling dead bodies. *Journal of Nervous and Mental Disorders, 178,* 396–398.

Weisaeth, L. (1983). *The study of a factory fire.* Unpublished doctoral dissertation, University of Oslo.

Weissberg, M. P., & Katz, T. A. (1991). The crash of Continental 1713: The impact on hospital-based personnel. *Journal of Emergency Medicine, 9,* 459–463.

Chapter 5

Group Psychotherapy for War-Related PTSD with Military Veterans

Julian D. Ford and Judith Stewart

Group psychotherapy with military veterans suffering from "war neurosis" was first reported shortly after World War II (Dynes, 1945). It was not until the early 1970s that groups were widely employed as a therapeutic modality with war veterans, primarily in the form of *rap groups* (Lifton, 1973; Shatan, 1973). Rap groups typically were leaderless, or were led by peers who viewed their role as that of a facilitator of honest and open emotional ventilation rather than as that of diagnostician or psychotherapist. The success of rap groups in providing the often grievously missing sense of homecoming and camaraderie was a significant factor in the United States government's unprecedented funding in 1979 of an entirely new branch of the Department of Veterans Affairs (VA)—the Readjustment Counseling Service and its program of more than 150 community-based Vet Centers.

However, rap groups were not able to resolve the complex and persistent problems of psychosocial readjustment experienced by many Vietnam veterans. In 1980 the American Psychiatric Association's Diagnostic and Statistical Manual (DSM-III) modified a longstanding position of viewing war (and other) trauma as having limited and transient psychosocial impact by codifying the diagnostic classification of post-traumatic stress disorder (PTSD). Several epidemiological investigations in the 1970s and 1980s demonstrated that as many as one in two military veterans who served in the Vietnam war zone experienced PTSD at some point since the war, documenting war-related PTSD's prevalence, severity, and chronicity. As the veterans themselves began to seek additional help for this highly refractory disorder, psychotherapists were called upon to develop counseling groups that preserved the open, intense and supportive sharing possible in rap groups while also providing frank psychotherapeutic treatment.

Early reports of psychotherapy groups with military veterans suffering from war zone PTSD were provided by clinicians working not only in the United States (Brende, 1981; Frick & Bogart, 1982; Walker & Nash, 1981) but also in Israel (Rosenheim & Elizur, 1977) and New Zealand (Boman, 1982). Two decades or more later, psychotherapy groups continue to be provided for military veterans by the Israeli Defense Forces (Solomon, Bleich, Shoham, Nardi, & Kotler, 1992), in Vietnam Veteran Counseling Service hospitals and outreach centers across Australia (Creamer, Jackson, & Ball, 1996), and in several hundred United States Department of Veterans Affairs (VA) programs—150 community-based Vet Centers, 190 outpatient mental health clinics, 100 hospital inpatient psychiatry units, and 125 specialized outpatient and inpatient PTSD programs. Women as well as men veterans of diverse ethnic and cultural backgrounds receive group psychotherapy for PTSD from all branches of military service and from eras ranging from World War II and the Korean war to as recently as the Persian Gulf war and United Nations peacekeeping operations in the 1990s.

WHAT RESEARCH EVIDENCE SUPPORTS THE USE OF GROUP PSYCHOTHERAPY WITH MILITARY VETERANS?

Controlled outcome research on the efficacy and cost-effectiveness of group therapy for PTSD with military veterans is virtually nonexistent. This lack is not surprising, given the paucity of data on group psychotherapy outcomes with any clinical population, but it bodes very poorly for the continued funding of group therapy in the present era of managed care and empirically validated treatment methods (Chambless et al., 1996).

A preliminary study by Ford and Mills (1995) compared two approaches to group therapy focused on helping veterans to emotionally process intrusive war trauma memories within an inpatient PTSD milieu treatment program. One method involved each veteran doing an extended (e.g., one or two consecutive group sessions) oral *walk through* to reprise chronologically his most disturbing or memorable pre-military, military training, war zone, and postwar experiences, with particular focus on war traumas. The alternative method, *guided trauma disclosure* (GTD), differed in two key ways. First, in order to enhance genuine cohesion based upon members' careful examination of personal differences and similarities, prewar and postwar experiences were reviewed in group discussion format, rather than as individual dissertations. Second, members selected, wrote, and (at the beginning of each of the sixth through twelfth sessions of the 18-session group) read and imaginally reexperienced a brief personal script describing a single war trauma memory in vivid sensory, affective, and cognitive detail. The trauma script readings and reimaginings were guided therapeutically to enhance the veteran's capacities for experiencing affect in a modulated fashion, reevaluating cognitive schemas for self, safety, and a just world, and reaching out and accepting social support. At a four-month follow-up, the GTD participants reported significantly lower PTSD symptoms on the PTSD Checklist and higher levels of self-esteem and satisfaction with work and intimacy on the Quality of Life Inventory than the walk-through group participants. Thus, trauma focus group therapy may be most beneficial when structured to emphasize participant psychosocial competence in dealing with trauma memories and PTSD symptoms, rather than as an expunging of all memories of trauma.

The VA's National Center for PTSD has launched a multisite controlled trial comparing a trauma-focused approach versus a social problem-solving variant of group psychotherapy with Vietnam veterans diagnosed with chronic PTSD (Friedman & Schnurr, 1995). The effects of each type of group will be assessed for six male veterans in 20 separate groups of each type over a follow-up period of a year after the conclusion of a set of 30 weekly outpatient sessions. Compared to Ford and Mills's GTD, a more prolonged form of therapeutic exposure to trauma memories is being used, but the protocol retains an emphasis upon gaining mastery with a single trauma memory and uses a homework self-exposure protocol adapted from GTD. The principal aim is to reduce the participating veterans' symptomatic severity and psychosocial impairment sufficiently so that they no longer warrant a PTSD diagnosis. In addition, the benefits of group therapy also will be assessed regarding the alleviation of severe depression, anxiety, dissociation, and alcohol and drug use problems associated with PTSD, and regarding the enhancement of each veteran's quality of work life, relationships, and self-esteem.

Several outcome evaluation studies have been reported for multimodal inpatient PTSD treatment programs in which group psychotherapy is a central component. These document mixed and at best weak positive gains (Fontana & Rosenheck, 1997; Ford, Fisher & Larson, 1997; Hammarberg & Silver, 1994; Hyer, Woods, Bruno & Boudewyns, 1989; Johnson et al., 1996; Munley, Bains, Frazee & Schwartz, 1994; Scurfield, Kenderdine & Pollard, 1990). Although it appears that some veterans benefit substantially from multimodal group-focused inpatient PTSD treatment (while others change little or even experience deterioration), no basis for clinically identifying the most appropriate candidates for these programs had been empirically validated until a recent study by Ford et al. (1997). That study described a reliable four-item protocol with which clinicians rate the capacity of each veteran to manage intense emotions and to maintain engagement in significant relationships—their *object relations*—and found these ratings could independently distinguish veterans whose PTSD (regardless of initial symptomatic severity) improved versus those whose PTSD did not change or worsened. These results, while based upon a multimodal program that included individual case management, counseling, and medication monitoring as well as group therapy, suggest that group psychotherapy may need to assess and treat not only PTSD symptoms but also each veteran's basic capacities for regulating emotion and engaging in relationships.

A study by Ragsdale, Cox, Finn, and Eisler (1996) called into question the benefits of group therapy with veterans when done independently of a multimodal treatment program. They found inpatient milieu treatment to be superior to ongoing outpatient group therapy (which had no discernable benefit) in improving veterans' hopelessness, loneliness, guilt, shame, and emotional expressiveness. However, neither freestanding group therapy nor the multimodal inpatient program reduced veterans' anger, anxiety, depression, relationship problems, or PTSD symptoms. Moreover, the veterans receiving group therapy were awaiting entry to specialized inpatient PTSD treatment, so it is unclear to what extent their failure to show positive changes was due to expectancies (e.g., belief that ordinary group therapy does not help, but special inpatient treatment does) rather than to any intrinsic deficiency in group therapy or any unique benefit of the inpatient milieu. The study does suggest that group therapy, whether done on an inpatient or outpatient basis, may be more effective if it is structured to provide a periodic *recharging* (e.g., revised goals or activities) rather than simply more of the same. Such a view is consistent with a recent study (Ronis et al., 1996) which showed that veterans in VA health care who are diagnosed with PTSD tend to engage in treatment episodically rather than continuously, alternating long periods of low utilization with bursts of intensive care.

Two studies of the process of group psychotherapy with military veterans suffering from PTSD have been reported. Scurfield et al. (1984–1985) had a participant observer sit in on 81 sessions of three groups over a nine-month period, noting the symptoms, personal issues, therapeutic themes, and therapist interventions occurring in each session. The groups tended to focus initially on highly emotional discussion of negative experiences in Vietnam and thereafter, largely directed by the veterans' spontaneous exclamations of anger, disillusionment, and distrust. Over a period of several sessions, the thematic focus shifted toward an emphasis upon intrusive reexperiencing symptoms (waking and in sleep), and a fear of losing control due to continuing feelings of rage and helplessness. Group members next shifted toward acknowledging and attempting to resolve previously unspoken problems of guilt, emotional emptiness and detachment from both relationships and productive involvement in work and community life.

Kanas, Schoenfeld, Marmar, Weiss, and Koller (1994) identified similar personal and therapeutic issues from therapist ratings of a group climate questionnaire over the course of a sequence of four 16-session blocks in an ongoing psychodynamic group therapy for veterans with PTSD. Compared to similar groups done with neurotic or schizophrenic members, the PTSD group sessions were rated as higher in cohesion and engagement and lower in avoidance or conflict. Clinical observation indicated, however, that the cohesion was superficial (Parson, 1985) because group members actually avoided rather than resolved intra- and interpersonal conflicts by adopting an *us against them* bonding based upon externalization of blame (i.e., diffuse rage and hopelessness regarding society and personal relationships). In contrast to the Scurfield et al. report and to similar studies of group therapy with other populations, as well as to clinical observations of group therapy for PTSD with veterans (see below), Kanas et al. detected no clear phasic progression in group climate or focal topics over time. However, this may be an artifact of the group essentially having to start anew every 16 sessions when participants took a two- to three-week break and often (>50%) dropped out and were replaced by new members. To facilitate group phasic progression and reduce premature terminations, the authors recommend providing pregroup orientation sessions, structured exercises at the start of each session, and a longer cycle (e.g., 20 to 25 sessions) or a continuous group without the artifice of regular breaks.

PRINCIPLES AND TECHNIQUES OF GROUP PSYCHOTHERAPY WITH MILITARY VETERANS

Group psychotherapy with military veterans serves several purposes through a variety of interventions which are conducted over a number of developmental phases in accord with key technical guidelines. We will review these considerations with illustrative case examples.

Purposes or Goals

Group psychotherapy enables military veterans to directly contravene the fundamental symptomatic binds of PTSD in carefully titrated doses of interpersonal (rather than isolated) engagement. In several unique ways, group therapy provides a safe place for ventilation of previously overwhelming emotions, for reconstructing healthy relationships, for regaining a sense of personal competence and meaning in life, and for reintegration into life and society.

Giving Testimony and Bearing Witness Group psychotherapy provides therapeutic boundaries (e.g., therapists have no hidden agendas and take responsibility for handling the effects of vicarious trauma), limits (e.g., violent feelings may be expressed but not acted upon), and a social sanction for ventilation of emotions that may otherwise be too terrifying or humiliating and for recounting of experiences that may otherwise lead to scapegoating and rejection (e.g., participation is reframed as a form of responsible self-care). The dual mandate of group psychotherapy—to enable each participant to access a livable truth while causing no harm to any person—facilitates a therapeutic reexperiencing, owning and letting go, and working through of terror, horror, shame, and loss by each veteran and (by proxy) on the part of the whole community and society that sent the soldier to war. The often voiced rageful demand for *payback*, which was drilled into most military personnel in training and in war, can be transmuted by bearing witness to a spiritual and existential renewal of the personal quest for fairness, justice, and compassion. Group discussion of each veteran's life story can restore the capacity for narrative memory and self-understanding that tends to be fragmented and shattered by war trauma, including a thorough and searching self-examination of how trauma has altered or complicated each member's core lifelong psychological dilemmas.

Revivification of Interpersonal Attachments   Although psychological trauma is an extreme form of existential and biological isolation, military personnel often experienced (or longed for the opportunity to do so) war trauma as a member of a team of peers who shared both the tragedy and the responsibility of the often overwhelming events. Psychotherapy groups can powerfully evoke this formative interpersonal aspect of war trauma in a context of current emotional safety and social support. Even if closely bonded with an emotionally secure team of comrades in arms, military personnel often report having felt completely alone and cut off emotionally, even from themselves when confronted with terror, help-lessness, or the moral and spiritual shock of exposure to "the evil that men do." Many war veterans served in roles purposefully detached from other soldiers or sailors—such as that of the officer, the medic or nurse, the tunnel rat, or the radio operator—and experienced war trauma as a necessary kind of exile from human-kind. Group involvement can be remoralizing and revivifying of a sense of a trusted community of people committed to healing not harming. Thus, returning to the team that was, or the team that never was but should have been, can provide a basis for reworking several therapeutic issues, including grieving the loss of camaraderie and innocence, confronting the contradiction of having felt invulner-able and yet powerless and shamed, facing the isolation of abandonment and betrayal, and confronting a terror of trust and intimacy.

Facing and Transmuting Terror, Rage, Guilt, and Shame   War trauma is profoundly alienating when death and devastation shatter or violate a soldier's sense of personal competence (e.g., "I went to pieces and froze under fire.") and worth (e.g., "I became a stone cold killer."). Life itself may seem to be pointless or without any meaningful future (e.g., "I should have died, I wish I had died, and I feel dead inside."). Nonjudgmental and reflective facilitation of group discussion of these intensely felt and believed reactions can provide an empathic validation of the universality of terror, rage, guilt, and shame as phenomenological sequelae of trauma—while simultaneously challenging the validity of associated scapegoating and stigmatization that veterans, unfortunately, often experienced since their homecoming in their relationships and in their self-appraisals. The group provides a supportive *holding environment* or *transitional space* (Winnicott, 1986) in which extreme and self-debilitating emotional and existential dilemmas can be examined with an emphasis upon honesty and healing rather than upon legal or moral blame and punishment. Group psychotherapy can assist veterans in facing emotions and schematic (often implicit) beliefs about themselves (e.g., self as monstrous or impoverished, full of hate or utterly empty) and their lives (e.g., perpetual abandonment and betrayal) that otherwise are too terrifying and humiliating to psychically come to terms with.

Regaining the Capacity for Initiative and Productivity   In light of the extreme existential despair perpetuated in chronic PTSD, it is not surprising that the sense of hope and motivation necessary for self-directed and productive involvement in work, education, recreation, and relationships is often severely diminished. Voicing externalized blame toward the government, the military, authorities, civilians, war protestors, or society in general often appears to be the PTSD veteran's sole (pre)occupation and reason for living. Explicit exhortations to engage in personally and socially responsible proactive planning and action often meet with responses of rage (e.g., "Why should I be a good citizen, when I've had my life ruined by a society that used me up and spit me out?") or passive resistance (e.g., "Why bother, when nothing ever gets any better and anything I do just seems to make things worse?"). Group psychotherapy can provide a direct experiential opportunity to experiment gradually with initiative (e.g., choosing when and about what to speak) in the context of a cooperative, rather than combative, sharing (rather than being entrapped and isolated) of responsibility, rather than blame. It can provide a context for solving problems, rather than feeling trapped by them, and achieving meaningful personal goals, rather than feeling manipulated and disenfranchised. Contributing as a member in group therapy thus noncoercively facilitates the in vivo resumption of self-initiated productive involvements in relationships and work that have direct personal significance and meaning.

Temporal and Developmental Phases

Over time, psychotherapy groups addressing PTSD progress through developmental phases paralleling the ontogeny of the person and the evolution of psychologically significant relationships. The Scurfield et al. (1984) and Kanas et al. (1994) studies provide helpful reminders that such phases are neither automatic, linear, nor universal. Indications that these phases are nonautomatic would be structural arrangements such as the scheduling of entry by new members, therapist attitudes and style, and group composition can short-circuit certain phases and prolong others. Indications that they are nonlinear are groups tend to revisit past themes and issues, and ways of interacting in cycles that are not necessarily predictable. Indications that they are nonuniversal are the many different themes and issues that characterize each unique group and its change over time. Nevertheless, several experienced clinicians have independently described parallel sets of developmental milestones and thematic foci characterizing groups with military veterans with PTSD (Brende, 1984; Frick & Bogart, 1982; Parson, 1988; Rosenheim & Elizur, 1977).

Selection and Preparation   Before entering a group, prospective members must be given an orientation and assessed for their readiness for the group and the group's appropriateness for them (Reaves & Maxwell, 1987; Trotta et al., 1990). The preparatory orientation consists of a description of the group's essential goals. These goals would include to assist in managing anger or stress and to deal with unresolved trauma memories from noncombat or combat military service. Also described during the orientation are relevant characteristics of current members. Thus, without violating confidentiality, the mix of gender, ages, and military backgrounds is described. Finally, the ground rules (such as commitment to attend on a regular basis while abstaining from substance use) are detailed. Offering a descriptive sample of how the group actually works in a session can debunk common preconceptions and give the veteran a tangible idea of how the group respects privacy and encourages individuality. For example:

> We begin and end each 90-minute session right on time (barring occasional emergencies), with a check-in in which each member says whatever they are comfortable sharing about how they're feeling and what's going on in their lives right at that moment and in the past and upcoming weeks. Each member also says if they want to take some time that session to talk over something at more length. The other group leader, who is a Vietnam in-country vet, and I don't try to psychoanalyze anyone, but we help the group to identify issues such as anger, loss, or frustration at work or in relationships. We try to help group members to get a handle on what's going right or wrong in their lives and what they may need to do to deal with life or PTSD in a way they feel is right for them.

Screening prospective participants usually involves several steps and sources. First, the group leader discusses the veteran's therapeutic status and issues with the therapist or case manager referring the veteran for group therapy. In the case of self-referral, an ongoing case management or individual therapy relationship is established (sometimes with a group leader serving in this role). The nature, frequency, and intensity of such one-to-one care will vary depending upon the veteran's individual psychosocial status, and it will change as the veteran's PTSD and associated psychological and medical health concerns stabilize, improve, or worsen. One-to-one psychosocial care is separated from group therapy in order to explicitly underscore the importance of the veteran having a mental health primary provider to ensure continuous and coordinated care, while enabling each veteran to use the group as a milieu for experimentation with self-expression, mutual support, and personal and relational problem-solving without any pressure or expectation of having to *fix* everything in group alone.

Second, screening includes assessing likely rule-outs for group psychotherapy in general, or this group in particular. Each group and group facilitator has different criteria, but the most common rule-outs for PTSD groups with veterans include the following conditions if not stable under current therapeutic management: mania, psychosis, substance abuse, recurrent emergency psychiatric or medical hospitalizations, or imminent suicidality. Veterans with chronic PTSD often have comorbid severe Axis I and Axis II disorders (Bremner, Southwick, Johnson, Yehuda, & Charney, 1993; Kulka et al., 1990) and physical health problems, or both (Friedman & Schnurr, 1995), which may require adjustments to the milieu in which group psychotherapy is done. For example, the therapy may be better in a day or partial hospitalization rather than outpatient context. The focus and goals of group psychotherapy may also need adjusting (e.g., emphasis may be better upon symptom management and here-and-now coping with life stressors rather than trauma memory exploration). Given the extremely high rates of comorbidity of chronic military-related PTSD and substance abuse, VA has developed a network of specialized VA outpatient and residential programs which provide an integrative rather than compartmentalized approach to treatment with a strong emphasis upon group interventions.

Encountering the Unendurable   When veterans first join PTSD psychotherapy groups, they, as individuals, and the group as a whole tend initially to focus on finding areas of common ground while struggling with intense feelings of distrust and fear of rejection or loss, as well as with a concomitant increase in emotional numbing and social detachment. Particularly in Vietnam, "f——ing new guys" tended to be viewed as liabilities whose inexperience placed themselves and their entire team at high risk for getting hurt or killed. The new guy's relative naivete and innocence also served as a poignant and painful reminder of the youthful emotional hopefulness and interpersonal vitality that war-torn warriors felt was irrevocably lost. The green new guy often felt overwhelmed and helpless in the face of the unprecedented demands and horrors of war, in addition to often having felt morally and physically violated and humiliated by his first introduction to the military in brutal and dehumanizing courses of basic and advanced training.

Thus, when veterans enter a group, both the ongoing and new members struggle with the revivification of the most intense feelings associated with military service and war (Frick & Bogart, 1982). Envy is mixed with contempt felt toward oneself as well as toward others. Shock, detachment, and rage manifest as precursors to intense grief. Profound alienation and hopelessness trigger regression (Rosenheim & Elizur, 1977) to primitive states of emotional numbing and detachment (Brende, 1984), narcissistic idealization and devaluation (Parson, 1985), and passive or aggressive social isolation. Angry declamations about the betrayals propagated by greedy, ruthless, and sadistic authorities, or about the stupidity and haplessness of civilians or other identified out-groups, tend to dominate the spontaneous interaction for several reasons. Verbalized rage serves as a defense against the twin terrors of annihilation—violent loss of control or demoralizing emotional numbing. Defining a common faceless evil adversary reenacts the depersonalization of the enemy necessary for many soldiers to tolerate killing, and establishes other group members as pseudofriends because of being "the enemy of my enemy." Hence the oft observed paradox of initial suspicious wariness cooccurring with an almost instantaneous identification with other group members as lost brothers and sisters, described by Parson (1988) as "prematurely accelerated cohesion."

The group leaders are very much in the midst of these powerful implicit currents of psychic terror and grief, and they are often faced with the direct fallout of primitive psychic splitting in the form of projective identification (e.g., "You're just here to keep us under control and to draw your government pay check.") or symbiotic enmeshment (e.g., "You're one of us, doc. You always know exactly what to say or do."). Therapeutic interventions at this early phase tend to mirror and reparatively clarify the unspoken emotional agendas in play. Straightforward and clear limits and boundaries are articulated calmly and empathically, framed as a way to make the group safe for all participants, e.g.,

> It's time to close today's session, and we need to be sure to continue to work together next session to find answers to the important questions several members have posed about whether you can trust this group and us as your leaders.

Integrative thematic foci are identified to help members gradually to relinquish the false security of pseudocohesion by finding a genuine basis for interpersonal bonding. This involves facilitating a recognition of how individual differences can coexist with a shared quest to rectify universal dilemmas such as abandonment, betrayal, loss of self-respect, helplessness, and loss of religious faith, and to recapture universal ideals like genuine courage, compassion, respectfulness, intimacy, and integrity as worthy contributions to a good society. The goal in this early phase is not to dispute or correct members' self-defeating behavior patterns, primitive defenses, or irrational beliefs, because these tend at this point to be experienced as an invalidation and to give rise to power struggles and acting out. Rather, leaders model integrity and respectfulness in the face of emotional chaos. They do so by setting limits consistent with members' own desires to achieve greater safety by gaining control of previously overwhelming impulses, and supporting each member's implicit goal of finding meaning, hope, and self-esteem in the struggle to live with the intense inner and relational turmoil of PTSD.

Giving Voice to the Unspeakable As members become able to define and discuss their current lives and their formative memories in terms of both highly individual circumstances and shared dilemmas, the group shifts almost imperceptibly into a phase of learning how to name and place into a coherent personal life history the unresolved emotional wounds of trauma. Issues that have been obscured by the fragmenting of consciousness in trauma become enacted in the interplay amongst group members and in their discussion of extragroup concerns. Death and dehumanization become foci as members describe how they have become both a killer and a victim (Brende, 1984). Underneath the rage, members help one another recognize and name feelings of profound despair, shame, survivor guilt, self-doubt, aloneness, and dependency (Parson, 1988; Rosenheim & Elizur, 1977). Members enact and then articulate the helpless sense of terror that has fueled years of subsequent hypervigilance and self-destructive attempts to test, and perhaps ultimately to disprove, their facade of invulnerability and indifference. As trust in the group, in the leaders, and in their own capacity to tolerate terror, shame, and despair grows, members may reveal atrocities that shattered their sense of a worthy self, a life to return to, a just world, and a guiding spiritual presence (Frick & Bogart, 1982).

Group leaders enable members to pay conscious attention to these previously unspoken and unspeakable emotional dilemmas and wounds. This is done by demonstrating experientially that it is possible to survive and gain a sense of mastery in encounters with trauma by carefully defining the personal significance of the suffering and by setting personally tolerable limits on what and how much the veteran chooses to remember or feel in each encounter. Leaders play a role paralleling that of Virgil in Dante's *Inferno*, guiding the weary and horrified journeyers by serving as the muse who gives meaning to the dreadful confrontation with their "sins," the traumas they've endured and the errors or impossible choices that they've made. Each "circle" of hell is akin to a deepening awareness of the emotional impact of trauma, and to the recognition of the crucial need to take responsibility for creating genuinely safer and healthier circumstances in their current lives, relationships, and communities.

As members take on this challenge, the group offers a unique holding environment of authentic respect and compassion. The therapeutic agenda is to assist each veteran in transmuting what has been an involuntary and utterly helpless repetition of senseless and indescribable, emotional annihilation, into a consciously initiated and deconstructed reexperiencing of understandable events and emotions. At some point(s) in the facing and naming of these unspeakable sorrows and humiliations, group members and leaders may become the target of inchoate rage or utter dependency, or both, emanating from a member who feels overwhelmed by despair or self-loathing (Frick & Bogart, 1982). The group leaders immediately step in, calmly but firmly bearing the brunt of the discharge, empathizing with the member's pain and dilemma, taking responsibility for helping the member to find a way to work through the crisis safely, and redefining the challenge as one of developing ways to experience and heal from pain without hurting self or other group participants.

Returning to the Previously Unreachable Future   With repeated experience in directly surviving the reexperiencing of what had been overwhelming distress due to traumatization and PTSD, and in witnessing and supporting peers in this process, group members tentatively begin to recognize and then to own a growing sense of returning from the dead. Increased self- esteem, autonomy, initiative, and motivation (Parson, 1985) emerge along with a capacity to feel both sorrow and hope (Brende, 1984). Rage, helplessness, and blame continue to be felt and expressed, but as preludes to examination of more vulnerable (e.g., grief, fear) and engaged (e.g., love, dedication) affects. Emotions are examined in relationship to current (and past) interpersonal involvement, and constructive social problem-solving ensues as a means to deal with issues such as intimacy, friendship, productivity, and personal self-care. Group leaders often become less overtly active in this phase, while remaining unobtrusively involved in a consultative role. They provide technical guidance about problem-solving, reminders about the principal themes and issues that link past traumatic (and other) experiences to current emotions and dilemmas, and a nonjudgmental source of emotional support and continuity.

Small Steps Toward Closure: Living with PTSD   When a group comes to a close and disbands, or if a veteran discontinues participation in an ongoing group, this termination typically does not signal the end of treatment for military-related PTSD. Veterans receiving care in the VA for PTSD tend to experience periods of therapy of differing degrees of intensity over many years, alternately in inpatient and outpatient settings, on frequent (e.g., weekly) or maintenance (e.g., bimonthly) bases (Ronis et al., 1996). A principal challenge to the group leader and each member is recognizing, anticipating, and managing the unavoidable resurgence of PTSD symptoms. The archetypal Greek myth explaining the seasons of the year fits the experience of many veterans with PTSD and of most PTSD therapy groups. Persephone, an innocent maiden, was kidnapped by the god of the underworld and taken into Hades. Although rescued by the love, courage, and perseverance of her mother Demeter, who simply refused to forget and abandon her daughter, once Persephone had been taken to Hades she was never fully free of its curse. Each year, Persephone must return to Hades for a time during which the whole world experiences the bleak colorlessness and chill of winter. Then she is freed temporarily to return to the world during the period of rebirth occurring in spring and summer. Like Persephone, youthful soldiers who lose their innocence in the hell of war can never, despite experiencing periods of renewal through the remoralization and dedication to healing provided in group psychotherapy, permanently escape the return to trauma and PTSD.

Just as group participation begins with a preparatory phase, so too does it come to a close with a second period of preparation—for life. Formally, therapeutic closure requires careful attention to relapse prevention, which involves anticipation and rehearsal of practical strategies for maintaining self-enhancing attitudes and activities and for coping effectively with temporary worsening of PTSD symptoms as well as of associated psychosocial problems (e.g., depression, urges to use substances, family conflict). Relapse prevention techniques are derived from sources as diverse as substance abuse treatment, systemic family therapy, and cognitive-behavioral therapy. The goal is to ensure that each veteran departs from group therapy with a psychological tool kit that includes resources to be called upon in a crisis; skills for managing stress, anger, and self-defeating habits; practical guidelines for expressing and making sense of emotions; skills for social communication and problem-solving; and a plan for pursuing meaningful goals via activities matched to the individual's interests and values.

Equally important, but somewhat less formulaic in actual practice, is the achievement of a sense of personal and relational closure by each group member. The personal side of closure involves bearing witness or giving testimony by articulating the key psychic themes and issues that describe in down-to-earth terms (a) how trauma and PTSD have changed the individual's life, and (b) the personal meaning and sense of self that the individual derives from surviving trauma and from mastering, but not eliminating, its sequelae (PTSD). The relational aspect of closure involves putting into practice a commitment to meaningful ongoing engagement in relationships (e.g., with primary partner, family members, friends, and group members). Achieving personal and relational closure can be facilitated by ritualized ceremonies such as a graduation in which members honor each other's participation and affirm their learning and commitments.

Special Issues

Practical Parameters   Psychotherapy groups for veterans with PTSD tend to meet on a regularly scheduled basis consistent with the treatment milieu and the group's composition and goals. Session length typically is fixed and ranges from one to two hours. Inpatient groups may meet several times weekly, but outpatient groups most often meet once weekly. Although some are designated explicitly as open attendance or drop-in groups, more often PTSD groups require regular attendance and invite new members to join only on a preplanned basis. Group size typically ranges from the minimum (usually five) sufficient to provide a heterogeneous core of committed participants to the maximum (usually eight to ten) permitting every member to gain individual recognition and giving the group sufficient time to address all pressing issues each session.

Group Composition   Beyond the commonality of having experienced trauma in military service, group members typically are quite diverse. Some groups specifically limit attendees to veterans of a particular era (e.g., World War II), ethnicity (e.g., Black or Native Americans), military specialty (e.g., officers; nurses; medics) or trauma type (e.g., POWs) (Boehnlein et al., 1993), in order to provide a psychologically sheltered space in which members can address traumagenic dynamics such as stigmatization or powerlessness. However, groups with members of diverse ages and eras, ethnicity, military specialties, and combat or noncombat traumas have been reported to be successful in part because members are challenged to find commonalties despite traditional differences or antagonisms (Jelinek, 1987). Younger and older veterans often find in each other a positive parental or filial role model. Noncombat veterans (e.g., transportation crews, radio operators, medical staff, or artillery crews) often find that the front line soldiers and sailors, who, they believe, devalue them as "rear echelon mother f——ers," spontaneously and gratefully validate the reality of noncombat traumas and the contribution that noncombat personnel played in keeping combatants alive. Bitter racial conflicts that were fueled by the horror of war and ethnic and cultural politics of past eras often can be aired and resolved for the first time in decades by veterans whose maturity enables them to recognize the importance of facing old biases and building person-to-person relationships.

Group Foci: Educative, Supportive/Expressive, or Trauma Exploration   Despite their many differences, therapy groups for military veterans with PTSD tend to utilize three basic formats. Psychoeducational groups (e.g., McWhirter & Liebman, 1988; Reilly, Clark, Shopshire, Lewis, & Sorensen, 1994) are highly structured with didactic aids (e.g., worksheets, audiovisual presentations) and behavioral exercises (e.g., role play simulations) that teach a defined topic or set of skills (e.g., anger or stress management or social communication) in a time-limited format (e.g., a series of 10 weekly sessions). Leader direction takes precedence over member interaction. Education groups can serve as a self- and clinician-screening to determine readiness and need for other types of group or alternative modalities of psychotherapy, as well as an orientation to the basic format and ground rules of group therapy.

Supportive/expressive groups—as successors to the Rap Group model (Brende, 1981; Rozynko & Dondershine, 1991)—facilitate interactive discussion of current relational and psychological (Frick & Bogart, 1982; Parson, 1988; Walker & Nash, 1981) issues related to PTSD, including an identification of critical themes linking formative past experiences (one subset of which are war traumas) with current concerns or impairment. Such groups tend to meet regularly with a closed membership, on either an ongoing or cyclic (e.g., Kanas et al., 1994) basis. Focal topics and session structure are relatively open-ended, defined primarily by (a) an opening and closing check-in from each member, (b) ground rules emphasizing mutual respect in service of thoughtful self-exploration, and (c) a content focus on the interaction of each participant's military experiences with significant personal and familial themes and roles.

Trauma exploration groups emphasize a detailed review by each member of key military and war trauma experiences. Trauma exploration usually is preceded by an examination of earlier developmental benchmarks and followed by a discussion of postwar psychosocial adjustment issues (Koller, Marmar, & Kanas, 1992). Such groups tend to utilize a format similar to that of their supportive/expressive counterparts, but more formally structure the main body of each session in order to ensure that all developmental phases (and especially the military and war trauma experiences) are reviewed in detail orally by each member. Hybrid *trauma process* (Ford & Mills, 1995) groups combining the features of both supportive-expressive and trauma exploration have been developed as adjuncts to more intensive *trauma focus* groups to enable members to discover, explore and decrease the continuing impact of military traumas on post-trauma functioning (Stewart, 1995). In such groups, structured analytic, experiential and process exercises are used to help members to (a) identify and alter behavioral or emotional trauma reenactments, and (b) practice methods of reducing involuntary reenactments.

Most psychotherapy groups with veterans utilize some blend of the psychoeducational and supportive/expressive modalities. The therapeutic guidance may be derived from several orientations, most often the cognitive-behavioral (e.g., Reilly et al., 1994), interpersonal (e.g., Reaves & Maxwell, 1987), or psychodynamic (Marmar, Weiss, & Pynoos, 1995) models. An interesting recent example are groups providing psychoeducation and supportive/expressive guidance from a variety of orientations for veterans experiencing a hallmark of PTSD, severe sleep disturbances (Brockway, 1987; Coalson, 1995; Thompson, Hamilton, & West, 1995).

Integration of Multiple Modalities Group psychotherapy with veterans suffering from PTSD rarely stands alone. Group therapy for PTSD typically occurs concurrently with one-to-one psychotherapy, medication monitoring, and case management, as well as with couples and family therapy. Ongoing outpatient group therapy must be integrated carefully with treatment (including other therapeutic groups) offered in episodes of inpatient or partial hospitalization. Over longer periods of time, group therapy must be sequenced so as to provide an efficient and effective contribution to the veteran's progressive recovery from PTSD. Optimally, group therapists will coordinate with, or at a minimum will monitor, each participant's medical care as well, especially for stress-related health problems, for which veterans with PTSD are at elevated risk.

The complex and often chronic nature of psychosocial impairment in veterans with military-related PTSD (Friedman & Rosenheck, 1994) necessitates the careful placement of group psychotherapy within a multidisciplinary continuum of care. A primary care model can facilitate comprehensive and timely care because a single primary clinician coordinates and monitors the delivery of a biopsychosocial treatment plan by a team of providers (Ford, Ruzek, & Niles, 1996). The primary clinician's role includes developing matches between the veteran's needs and appropriate groups over the course of treatment. For example, psychoeducational groups with specific limited goals that maximize the chances of a positive response provide the veteran newly entering mental health care with a sample of the culture and potential of group therapy, while also providing the clinician with an assessment of the veteran's readiness for supportive/expressive group therapy. Supportive/expressive groups can accomplish a further assessment by and for the veteran, aiding in decisions about the appropriateness and timing of yet more intensive interventions such as trauma exploration groups or milieu treatment.

Addressing Comorbid Axis I Disorders An integrated continuous treatment plan is necessary to effectively provide group therapy when PTSD is complicated by comorbid disorders such as depression, substance dependency, or panic disorder. Veterans in group therapy for PTSD often describe reluctance to engage in other mental health modalities (e.g., alcoholism recovery programs or support groups). This may be based upon a fear, sometimes derived from actual experience, that their PTSD will be ignored or discounted (e.g., "The counselor told me PTSD is just an excuse and wouldn't help me figure out how to deal with urges to drink that happen when I feel like I'm back in Nam again."). Helping veterans accept that Axis I comorbid diagnoses are not unusual and are treatable is essential, as is fostering understanding of how comorbid conditions interact with the PTSD (e.g., activation of trauma triggers resulting in substance use lapses). Attention to Axis I comorbid disorders is not mutually exclusive with validation of trauma-specific symptoms and impairment. The reciprocally interactive nature of these problems means that neither is more or less important to the veteran's therapy.

Addressing Comorbid Axis II Features Characterological problems, such as grandiosity and devaluation, splitting and projective identification, passive-aggressiveness or dependency, and antisocial tendencies are both grist for the group therapeutic mill and potential major impediments to effective group psychotherapy. Although veterans in PTSD treatment have elevated rates of personality disorder diagnoses (Bremner et al., 1993), most do not qualify for Axis II diagnoses and therefore group therapists should not assume that extreme characterologic problems will be the norm. A substantial proportion of veterans in treatment for extremely debilitating chronic PTSD show evidence of quite positive characterological capacities, despite often struggling with severe emotional dysregulation and interpersonal alienation (Ford et al., 1997). The relatively rare extreme manifestations of characterological dysfunction (e.g., parasuicidal self-harm, dissociative identity disturbance, uncontrolled rage) are very disruptive in most veteran PTSD groups and probably better treated within a milieu or program specifically structured to place PTSD issues secondary to enhancing the capacity to safely participate in treatment (e.g., dialectic behavior therapy, partial hospitalization).

War trauma experienced in late adolescence or early adulthood (often compounded by demoralizing or even traumatic prewar military training) appears to leave an indelible biopsychosocial imprint of terror, horror, guilt and shame, unresolved grief, betrayal, abandonment, spiritual alienation, and profound identity confusion or self-loathing. Even in the absence of childhood traumatization or behavior problems, these complex post-traumatic sequelae can cause veterans who are characterologically resilient to experience severe episodic struggles with Axis-II-like symptoms (e.g., rage, emptiness, isolation) consistent what have been called "Disorders of Extreme Stress" (Ford, 1999; Newman, Orsillo, Herman, Niles, & Litz, 1995). Groups offer opportunities to address simultaneously PTSD and these additional alterations in the regulation of emotion and consciousness. Groups marry the benefits of the therapeutic alliance with those of peer support and experiential learning, in three key ways:

1   by experiencing (to the extent tolerable) and understanding the specific emotion(s) and thoughts being activated (e.g., grief and loneliness embedded within a global sense of rage or despair);

2   by identifying trauma-related "triggers" (e.g., anniversary dates or current experiences that revive trauma memories or feelings); and

3   by making a plan to cope consciously and actively by being aware of the significance of the triggers, the normalcy of the emotions, and the specific immediate steps that will provide positive social support and an enhanced sense of self-respect and personal accomplishment.

Gender and Sexual Issues   Women veterans have tended to be forgotten warriors. Until quite recently they have been provided far fewer health services than men by the military or VA and much less acclaim by our society. The reasons for this are diverse but clear. There is a sense of marginalization where women who have served in the military are concerned, this despite the fact that they have been in the midst of clearly traumatizing experiences. The factors which contribute to marginalization may vary from era to era, yet have persisted for as long as women have served in the military. Societal marginalization results in a disconnection of the woman from her sense of herself as a veteran. Not only society in general and the military, but also healthcare providers, have been a source of this problematic psychic disconnection.

Women war-zone veterans often served as healthcare personnel, officers who were charged with caring for the wounded as in Vietnam. In this status, they experienced complex role requirements. They simultaneously cared for a stream of horribly wounded male casualties most of whom were younger than themselves, while themselves being restricted from carrying weapons. Many of these women experienced combat conditions, such as being overrun by enemy forces or need-ing to protect themselves from incoming fire. Their nursing experiences often are difficult, troubling and outside the range ever seen in civilian conditions (e.g., 500 amputations in a day; seeing a continual stream of 18- and 19-year-olds maimed and crippled), constituting a powerful variation of traumatic exposure to combat.

Women also serve in other capacities in the war zone (e.g., intelligence, trans-portation, communication), a trend which became the norm in the Gulf War. With this expansion of duties, many women in the military assumed positions of au-thority over male combatants in the war zone. Whether as intelligence officers or communications or transportation specialists, women have experienced not only combat equivalent to that of their male counterparts but also significant social and institutional pressures and discrimination. Moreover, where the Vietnam era was marked by a cohort of women who were fairly homogeneous (e. g., officer status, noncombatant positions), the Gulf War produced a cohort of women who are themselves heterogeneous, and who have experienced a wider scope of trau-matic war-zone events.

Yet another nuance often emerges in dealing with women veterans who seek treatment for war-related trauma. This is the experience of sexual harassment or sexual assault, often at the hands of military superiors or peers. Active duty sexual harassment and assault, particularly of female recruits by superiors while in early training stages, appears to have been a pervasive and long-standing problem despite only recently becoming highly profiled. Sexual harassment and assault in any context can constitute a traumatic threat to a woman's effectiveness and abil-ity to function. Unfortunately, sexual assault perpetrated by military personnel often occurs within the war zone, gravely compounding the already substantial trauma of combat exposure. The woman is confronted by profoundly conflicting senses of self. She is a combatant or a nurse, at times an officer, who is sent to the war zone to defend her country or administer to the wounded, and yet those on whom she depends for her survival, or for whom she is supposed to care, turn on her and perpetrate sexual violence against her. This betrayal (Freyd, 1994) and the resultant inability to integrate these senses of self leave many of these women veterans in a psychic state of limbo: confused, terrified, outraged at the violation, and filled with rage at themselves since they, by definition, are supposed to be the caregivers and protectors of others. These women veterans of course are not re-sponsible for the trauma of war or sexual abuse, but instead are seeking some way to understand the betrayal they've experienced with some sense of personal con-trol, even if this is achieved by self-blame.

Coming into treatment, women veterans must begin a series of reconnections with disconnected parts of themselves. They must reconnect with aspects of their own functioning as outlined above, so that, for example, rather than numbing in the face of strong dysphoric emotions elicited by some interpersonal interaction, they acknowledge the emotions and continue to engage with others. They often need to reclaim the sense of being a veteran, of having served their country, of deserving recognition, and of deserving psychological and medical treatment, whether it be for enemy-inflicted or friendly-inflicted traumatically damaging experiences. For many, there needs to be reconnection of their veteran selves with their positions in society. For many women, the military experience is stored in memory as a harrowing experience, and they keep it hidden from current civilian contemporaries.

This understanding of the experience of women veterans informs several choices about group treatment. Given the marginalization and disconnection which traumatized women veterans feel, therapeutic groups exclusively for and by women have particular value as safe places in which peers can join together to create an atmosphere which facilitates the recognition and reparation. By contrast, if women veterans are asked or required to join groups with male veterans, the historical role relationship of silent handmaiden to the wounded male is likely to be reinstated in the present. Moreover, a sexual assault survivor who is placed in a group with men working on war trauma (however well-intentioned and facilitated) is very likely to involuntarily (as opposed to therapeutically) revivify a traumatic sense of entrapment and vulnerability to male rage, violence, and betrayal.

As a result, not only have women veterans understandably been reluctant to seek health or psychological care within the VA system, but when they do so they tend to have difficulty finding appropriate services. Psychotherapy groups for women veterans suffering PTSD were almost nonexistent even in most VA hospitals or clinics (Buechler, 1992), although some were provided by the Vet Centers whose staff included female counselors. In the past decade, activism by women veterans has led to several encouraging developments in health care and psychotherapy. VA has established a central office for Women's Health Affairs, and Women Veterans' Health Clinics in dozens of VA hospitals or clinics, Women's Stress Disorder Treatment programs have been established at VA hospitals across the country, supported by a Women's Health Sciences Division of the VA National Center for PTSD, and VA's Readjustment Counseling Service has funded Vet Center staff positions dedicated to sexual trauma counseling.

Psychotherapy groups now are available specifically for women veterans in every area of the country. The Women's Trauma Recovery Program at the National Center for Post-traumatic Stress Disorder at the Palo Alto VA Health Care System has produced models for both inpatient and outpatient group treatment for military-related trauma (Stewart & De Angelo, 1997). These treatment models share many of the structural characteristics described throughout this chapter. The multimodal inpatient program is integrative and sequential in nature. It is milieu-based with most of the psychotherapeutic work occurring in the group format, since a core tenet of the treatment is that the ability of the traumatized veteran to reconnect with others (e.g., trust, accept confrontation feedback, and identify with others) is critical to the treatment of PTSD. Prior to admission, all referrals are screened to rule out conditions (e.g., Axis I and Axis II comorbidities or acute substance abuse) that would make group work difficult or impossible for the veteran. The veteran's capacity to tolerate intense emotions and to maintain engagement in relationships is also assessed as far as possible from written referral material. Inpatient treatment is scheduled (rather than on a crisis basis) and of sufficient length to permit women patients to develop a genuine working alliance with one another and with therapists. The sequencing of the program is purposeful, aimed at working towards the development of safety by the individual woman within the milieu (Herman, 1992).

Milieu-based inpatient treatment for women veterans does not pathologize the patient by focusing upon (presumptive) psychological deficits, but instead seeks to assist each woman in reconnecting the aspects of her self through experiencing the safety and understanding possible in a therapeutic community. Groups provide the vehicle for facilitating an initial entry into the milieu: for gradual experimentation with personal reflection and disclosure; for learning or the renewal of skills in stress management, anger and affect management, problem-solving, and interpersonal and intimate communication; and for individually-paced and designed exploration, within a focus psychotherapy group, of trauma within the military and its aftermath.

The final weeks of inpatient treatment are dedicated to a unique process of self-exploration and working-through within a lifespan perspective (Stewart, 1995). This involves a complete intensive emotional and cognitive reprocessing of significant life events emphasizing those which have been traumatic. The aim is the construction of a generative life narrative—a visual lifescript—that graphically highlights each woman's trauma experiences and their developmental impacts, and the triggers and patterns of reenactment that have perpetuated and exacerbated their disconnection from self and others. These disconnections often originated with sexual as well as war trauma, including a sense of being disconnected from the self (e.g., saying that things are "okay" when in fact they are enraged), from the self as a veteran (e.g., having service in the war zone completely eclipsed by the fact that rape also occurred), from the self and others (e.g., isolation and alienation from relationships which are more typically expected and accomplished by women, such as with their children), and society (e.g., strained relations with strangers and a sense that they do not fit in anywhere because of their experiences). The group assists each woman in reclaiming awareness and control in her life by creating this narrative lifescript. A final technique for reconnection is a group project that concretizes the patients' joint work in the tangible form of a panel for a quilt connecting each group to all prior ones and to those who follow.

An outpatient group was developed for women veteran war-zone trauma survivors who were not experiencing symptoms sufficient to necessitate hospitalization. Their subjective war-related experiences tended toward avoidance and numbing, and a sense of feeling that some aspect of their life experience was affecting their daily lives but without their conscious awareness of it. For example, they might experience days of feeling sad and thinking of the precarious nature of life, rather than a flood of intrusions related to the young casualties they had nursed). The group was a structured process group, which incorporated exercises aimed at life-review (Stewart, 1995) with a process aimed at the sharing of current experiences which appeared to have taken root in war-related experiences. In addition to regular weekly sessions, the group, leaders and members, traveled to Washington, D.C., for the unveiling of the Women's War Memorial, which provided a powerful experience of reconnection for the women with their veteran status.

Although the group did not specifically focus on war, military, or other trauma, most group members were able to face and achieve a sense of resolution with these memories. One member, became flooded by graphic intrusive recollections and requested an intensification of trauma work which she was able to pursue within the inpatient setting. With the support of the outpatient group, this woman was able to identify ways in which she had been devaluing herself as weak or deficient because of her continuing difficulty with intrusive symptoms, and to accept that the safety provided by the inpatient milieu was necessary for her to complete the more intensive trauma-focused work needed. This example illustrates the general guideline that intensive trauma focus group work with women veterans is often best done in an inpatient (or residential) milieu, while outpatient group work nevertheless can be sufficient to permit the working through of serious but less severe post-traumatic impairment.

Secondary Gain and Entitlement   Veterans may feel that they are placed in a bind when seeking treatment. They want to get help and improve their functioning, and yet in order to be eligible for PTSD treatment, they often must be judged to be disabled. If the disability improves as result of successful engagement in treatment, they may lose financial assistance and treatment eligibility before they are fully prepared to do without these supports. PTSD has a cyclical and fluctuating course, so improvement does not assure freedom from significant periods of symptomatic worsening (e.g., on dates that are trauma anniversaries or when other life stressors worsen). Veterans in group psychotherapy for PTSD often struggle with the dilemma of whether they can afford to feel better or make positive lifestyle changes which may place them at risk of losing access to a valued safety net while they are still vulnerable to PTSD's symptoms. Yet, for many veterans in group treatment, the idea of reliance upon the government or of getting social or health benefits is an anathema that contradicts a strong belief in self-reliance and in paying one's own way.

We have found that group treatment is most effective if veterans are helped to talk about their complex multivalenced reactions to disability and benefits explicitly, examining these as therapeutic issues rather than as guilty or shameful secrets. Although it is essential to establish that group therapy is not intended to help members get or keep disability benefits, the internal and interpersonal challenges involved in disability and benefits are vehicles for productive therapeutic work on coping, stress, anger, self-esteem, and relationships. Thus the focus can be shifted from unproductive attempts to externalize blame (e.g., political corruption, institutional failures) to a mutually-supportive reflection upon the underlying emotions (e.g., abandonment, shame, loss) and sources of resiliency and responsibility (e.g., personal values; family commitments) that otherwise are obscured by an externalized focus on entitlement.

Transference and Countertransference Strong interpersonal forces arise in the course of group psychotherapy with military veterans (Lindy & Wilson, 1994). For example, group members may view group leaders as first lieutenants, namely therapists who do therapy in a mechanical and detached manner ("by the book"), or as a brother or sister, namely persons with whom they feel so emotionally connected that it seems the leaders actually have shared their trauma experiences. Leaders may be viewed as authority figures who are burned out themselves (e.g., head nurses who drank to ease the pain of being in the war zone).

Such tranferences derive from group members' basic human need to achieve safety, relatedness, and mastery in the face of overwhelming emotions that are intensified, but not fundamentally caused by psychological trauma. Group therapy can help veterans to understand how these powerful transferential emotions and beliefs developed both through formative developmental experiences before the military and in highly emotionally charged role-relationships in the military involving traumatic abuse or war events. Thus, the fear and trepidation of the young officer who knew much from his studies but little of actual battle experiences can be examined through the therapist who acknowledges no combat experience, but knowledge and skill in treating trauma and deep caring for the welfare of the veteran. Or a nurse may be able to understand her conflicted response of hurt and dependency in relation to a harsh and distant head nurse, as group therapy enables her to acknowledge and rework her own absence of empathy when she derogated and condemned herself for having felt emotionally overwhelmed in the war zone. Group psychotherapy provides a forum in which veterans can recognize and make new choices in response to transferential dilemmas, rather than continuing to play them out in relationally and symptomatically debilitating manners.

Groups for male veterans often involve a female cotherapist. This affords members the opportunity to identify and resolve gender issues embedded in war trauma (Wakefield & Hyland, 1988). For example, war may involve the traumatic witnessing of or participating in killing of women, resulting in profound guilt, shame, and emotional numbing. The veteran may feel unable to reveal or even consciously retain awareness of these memories and feelings. As a consequence, the veteran may experience severe social detachment or rage, especially in relationships with women (or female children). Given this pattern, the male veteran may have experienced in his post-trauma life repeated abandonment by females when he begins to express his complex emotional feelings (e.g., rage and rejection of interpersonal connection), thus reinforcing for the male veteran his rejection by those, namely women, whom he has transgressed against during the war. A female cotherapist's presence can activate emotions associated with this gender-focused conflict. The female therapist's reactions and interventions can help the veteran to process complex feelings, and can begin to interact the blanket categorization of women as victims or emotional abandoners. The pairing of a male and female cotherapy team provides opportunities for role modeling (e.g., the male and female cotherapists' supportive and respectful interaction) and therapeutic guidance to assist the veteran in recognizing and resolving the emotional and relational impact of these buried traumas.

Countertransferential reactions are equally important. It is difficult for a female therapist to sit and listen to the detailing of the brutalizing of a female in the war zone, despite sound training and an understanding of how such acts by men against women could occur. Similarly when working with women veterans, there can be very strong reactions to hearing about the sexual harassment and assaults which are perpetrated by male soldiers on their female counterparts. For female therapists there may be identification with the wish to avenge the survivor, and for the male therapist a wish to discount or distance himself from either the abhorrence of perpetration or the vulnerability of the survivor. The power of the material disclosed in group work necessitates ongoing cotherapist processing of reactions, as well as an in-depth understanding of the interaction patterns of the group system.

CONCLUSION

There is a long tradition of using group psychotherapy for men and women who have been traumatized. Throughout history the need to talk about and process with others experiences of trauma has been central to healing psychic wounds. However, the advent of industrialization in the nineteenth century shifted the focus from a reintegration of trauma survivors back into society to the eradication of symptoms. In the past decade, neurobiological and cognitive science has demonstrated that traumatic stress creates lasting, not transient or eradicable, physiological and psychological changes. The intense, often prolonged, and also often morally and spiritually wounding trauma of war or sexual assault is particularly likely to have chronic sequelae, as do other traumatic experiences that involve prolonged vulnerability and violation. On the part both of the survivor and the psychotherapist, acceptance of a changed state is essential. However, acceptance is not tantamount to resignation or stigmatization.

Group treatment for military veteran survivors of war and sexual trauma thus aims not to cure PTSD, but to help each individual regain connection to (a) a sense of self that integrates experiences before, during, and after the military, and (b) personal, familial, and societal resources as a member of a safe and supportive community. Group therapy draws on the synergistic power of therapeutic guidance and peer relationships to assist each member in reconstructing a personal narrative that integrates trauma and powerlessness with a new sense of personal control and mutual support. Group work provides opportunities for interaction with not only fellow survivors but also those who have experienced other kinds of trauma and with untouched witnesses. Group therapy for military-related trauma thus frees members and leaders alike to fully recognize the lasting and profound impact of trauma, while exploring the potential for sharing little-by-little the experience of renewal.

REFERENCES

Boman, B. (1982). The Vietnam veteran ten years on. *Australian and New Zealand Journal of Psychiatry, 16,* 107–127.

Bremner, J. D., Southwick, S. M., Johnson, D. R., Yehuda, R., & Charney, D. S. (1993). Childhood physical abuse and combat-related post-traumatic stress disorder in Vietnam veterans. *American Journal of Psychiatry, 150,* 235–239.

Brende, J. O. (1981). Combined individual and group therapy for Vietnam veterans. *International Journal of Group Psychotherapy, 31,* 367–378.

Brende, J. O. (1984). An educational-therapeutic group for drug and alcohol abusing combat veterans. *Journal of Contemporary Psychotherapy, 14,* 122–136.

Brockway, S. S. (1987). Group treatment of combat nightmares in post-traumatic stress disorder. *Journal of Contemporary Psychotherapy, 17,* 270–284.

Buechler, D. (1992). Bringing together women Vietnam veterans. *NCP Clinical Newsletter, 2,* pp. 7, 10, & 18.

Coalson, R. (1995). Nightmare help: Treatment of trauma survivors with PTSD. *Psychotherapy, 32,* 381–388.

Dynes, J. B. (1945). Rehabilitation of war casualties. *War Medicine, 7,* 32–35.

Fontana, A., & Rosenheck, R. (1997). Effectiveness and cost of the inpatient treatment of post-traumatic stress disorder: Comparison of three models of treatment. *American Journal of Psychiatry, 154,* 758–765.

Ford, J. D., & Mills, P. (1995). *Guided trauma disclosure in the psychotherapy of chronic PTSD.* Paper presented at the Annual ISTSS Convention, Boston.

Ford, J. D. (1999). Disorders of extreme stress following war-zone military trauma. *Journal of Consulting and Clinical Psychology, 67,* 3–12.

Ford, J. D., Fisher, P., & Larson, L. (1997). Object relations as a predictor of treatment outcome with chronic PTSD. *Journal of Consulting and Clinical Psychology, 65,* 547–559.

Ford, J. D., Ruzek, J., & Niles, B. (1996). Identifying and treating VA medical care patients with undetected sequelae of psychological trauma and post-traumatic stress disorder. *NCP Clinical Quarterly, 6,* 77–82.

Freyd, J. J. (1994). Betrayal trauma: Traumatic amnesia as an adaptive response to child-hood abuse. *Ethics and Behavior, 4*, 307–329.

Frick, R., & Bogart, L. (1982). Transference and countertransference in group therapy with Vietnam veterans. *Bulletin of the Menninger Clinic, 46*, 429–444.

Friedman, M. J., & Schnurr, P. (1995). The relationship between trauma, post-traumatic stress disorder, and physical health. In M. J. Friedman, D. S. Charney, & A. Y. Deutch (Eds.), *Neurobiological and clinical consequences of stress: From normal adaptation to post-traumatic stress disorder* (pp. 507–524). Philadelphia: Lippincott-Raven.

Friedman, M. J., & Schnurr, P. P. (1995). *Group treatment of PTSD: VA cooperative study 420.* White River Junction, VT: National Center for PTSD.

Friedman, M., & Rosenheck, R. (1996). PTSD as a chronic disorder. In S. Soreff (Ed.), *The seriously and persistently mentally ill* (pp. 369–389). Seattle: Hogrefe & Huber.

Galloucis, M., & Kaufman, M. E. (1988). Group therapy with Vietnam veterans: A brief review. *Group, 12*(2), 85–102.

Hammarberg, M., & Silver, S. (1994). Outcome of treatment for post-traumatic stress disorder in a primary care unit serving Vietnam veterans. *Journal of Traumatic Stress, 7,* 195–216.

Herman, J. (1992). Complex PTSD. *Journal of Traumatic Stress, 5,* 377–391.

Hyer, L., Woods, M., Bruno, B., & Boudewyns, P. (1989). Treatment outcomes of Vietnam veterans with PTSD and the consistency of the MCMI. *Journal of Clinical Psychology, 45,* 547–552.

Jelinek, J. M. (1987). Group therapy with Vietnam veterans and other trauma victims. In T. Williams (Ed.), *Post-traumatic stress disorders: A handbook for clinicians* (pp. 209–219). Cincinnati, OH: Disabled American Veterans.

Johnson, D. R., Rosenheck, R., Fontana, A., Lubin, H., Charney, D., & Southwick, S. (1996). Outcome of intensive inpatient treatment for combat-related post-traumatic stress disorder. *American Journal of Psychiatry, 153,* 771–777.

Kanas, N., Schoenfeld, F. B., Marmar, C. R., Weiss, D. S., & Koller, P. (1994). Process and content in a long-term PTSD therapy group for Vietnam veterans. *Group, 18,* 78–88.

Koller, P., Marmar, C. R., & Kanas, N. (1992). Psychodynamic group treatment of post-traumatic stress disorder in Vietnam veterans. *International Journal of Group Psychotherapy, 42,* 225–246.

Kulka, R. A., Schlenger, W. E., Fairbank, J. A., Hough, R. L., Jordan, B. K., Marmar, C. R., & Weiss, D. S. (1990). *Trauma and the Vietnam War generation: Report of findings from the National Vietnam Veterans Readjustment Study.* New York: Brunner/Mazel.

McWhirter, J. J., & Liebman, P. C. (1988). A description of anger-control therapy groups to help Vietnam veterans with post-traumatic stress disorder. *Journal for Specialists in Group Work, 13*(1), 9–16.

Munley, P., Bains, D., Frazee, J., & Schwartz, L. (1994). Inpatient PTSD treatment. *Journal of Traumatic Stress, 7,* 319–325.

Newman, E., Orsillo, S., Herman, D., Niles, B., & Litz, B. (1995). Clinical presentation of disorders of extreme stress in combat veterans. *Journal of Nervous and Mental Disease, 183,* 628–632.

Parson, E. R. (1985). Post-traumatic accelerated cohesion: Its recognition and management in group treatment of Vietnam veterans. *Group, 9,* 10–23.

Parson, E. R. (1988). The unconscious history of Vietnam in the group: An innovative multiphasic model for working through authority transferences in guilt-driven veterans. *International Journal of Group Psychotherapy, 38,* 275–301.

Ragsdale, K. G., Cox, R. D., Finn, P., & Eisler, R. M. (1996). Effectiveness of short-term specialized inpatient treatment for war-related post-traumatic stress disorder: A role for adventure-based counseling and psychodrama. *Journal of Traumatic Stress, 9,* 269–283.

Reaves, M. E., & Maxwell, M. J. (1987). The evolution of a therapy group for Vietnam veterans on a general psychiatry unit. *Journal of Contemporary Psychotherapy, 17,* 22–33.

Reilly, P. M., Clark, H. W., Shopshire, M. S., Lewis, E. W., & Sorensen, D. J. (1994). Anger management and temper control: Critical components of post-traumatic stress disorder and substance abuse treatment. *Journal of Psychoactive Drugs, 26,* 401–407.

Ronis, D., Bates, E., Garfein, A., Buit, B., Falcon, S., & Liberzon, I. (1996). Longitudinal patterns of care for patients with post-traumatic stress disorder. *Journal of Traumatic Stress, 9,* 763–781.

Rosenheim, E., & Elizur, A. (1977). Group therapy for traumatic neuroses. *Current Psychiatric Therapies, 17,* 143–148.

Rozynko, V., & Dondershine, H. E. (1991). Trauma focus group therapy for Vietnam veterans with PTSD. *Psychotherapy, 28,* 157–161.

Scurfield, R. M., Kenderine, S. K., & Pollard, R. J. (1990). Inpatient treatment for war-related post-traumatic stress disorder: Initial findings on a longer-term outcome study. *Journal of Traumatic Stress, 3,* 185–201.

Scurfield, R. M., Teena, M., Gongla, P. A., & Hough, R. L. (1984). Three post–Vietnam "rap/therapy" groups: An analysis. *Group, 8,* 2–18.

Shatan, C. F. (1973). The grief of soldiers: Vietnam combat veterans' self–help movement. *American Journal of Orthopsychiatry, 43,* 640–653.

Smith, J. R. (1985). Rap groups and group therapy for Viet Nam veterans. In S. M. Sonnenberg, A. S. Blank, & J. A. Talbott (Eds.), *The trauma of war: Stress and recovery in Viet Nam veterans* (pp. 165–191). Washington, DC: American Psychiatric Press.

Solomon, S. D., Gerrity, E. T., & Muff, A. M. (August 5, 1992). Efficacy of treatments for post-traumatic stress disorder: An empirical review. *Journal of the American Medical Association, 268,* 633–638.

Solomon, Z., Bleich, A., Shoham, S., Nardi, C., & Kotler, M. (1992). The "Koach" project for treatment of combat-related PTSD: Rationale, aims, and methodology. *Journal of Traumatic Stress, 5,* 175–193.

Southwick, S. M., Yehuda, R., & Giller, E. L. (1993). Personality disorders in treatment-seeking combat veterans with post-traumatic stress disorder. *American Journal of Psychiatry, 150,* 1020–1023.

Stewart, J. (1995). Reconstruction of self: Life-span-oriented group psychotherapy. *Journal of Constructivist Psychology, 8,* 129–148.

Stewart, J., & De Angelo, D. (1997). *Women and military-related trauma: Experiences, impact and treatment strategies.* Manuscript submitted for publication.

Task Force on Promotion and Dissemination of Psychological Procedures. (1995). Training empirically-validated psychological treatments. *The Clinical Psychologist, 26,* 3–23.

Thompson, K. E, Hamilton, M., & West, J. A. (Fall 1995). Group treatment for nightmares in veterans with combat-related PTSD. *NCP Clinical Quarterly, 5*(4), 13–17

Trotta, F., Daniels, N., Stone, A., Gamble, G., Decatur, R., Mazarek, A., Gariti, K. O., Orton, G., Smith, M., Delmaestro, S., & Ternes, J. (December 1990). An orientation to PTSD therapy for combat veterans. *VA Practitioner, 7,* 69–71.

Wakefield, K., & Hyland, J. M. (January 1988). The importance of a female therapist in a male Vietnam veterans' psychotherapy group. *Bulletin of the Menninger Clinic, 52,* 16–29.

Walker, J. I., & Nash, J. L. (1981). Group therapy in the treatment of Vietnam combat veterans. *International Journal of Group Psychotherapy, 31,* 379–389.

Wilson, J. P, & Lindy, J. D. (1994). *Countertransference in the treatment of PTSD.* New York: Guilford Press.

Chapter 6

Psychological Treatment of Motor Vehicle Accident Survivors with PTSD: Current Knowledge and Application to Group Treatment

Edward J. Hickling and Edward B. Blanchard

This chapter outlines the known literature on the treatment of motor vehicle accident (MVA) survivors, reviews the treatment of MVA related post-traumatic stress disorder (PTSD), and concludes with a description of a piloted program conducted at the Albany MVA Treatment Project. To our knowledge, there has not been any group treatment for this population. It is important for the reader to understand that principles put forth in this chapter have been applied only for individual treatment. The treatment for MVA-related PTSD is clearly an emerging area and one where it is reasonable that application of individual treatment to group process could occur. This chapter, we believe, outlines those principles and applications that can be applied to group treatment. There is, however, a need for empirical evidence to support this belief. The reader, once again, is cautioned that this section has come exclusively from our knowledge based on individual treatment although we believe it can be very easily extrapolated to a group intervention. This chapter reviews the available information on treatment for PTSD following an MVA, and where possible, draws a parallel for group treatment.

Motor vehicle accidents are a widespread event in the United States, and much of the industrialized world. While precise data are not available, in the United States more than 3 million people suffer personal injuries as a result of an MVA and over 41,000 deaths were attributed to MVAs (Dept. of Transportation, 1995). A recent large-scale survey by Kessler, Sonnega, Brobet, Hughs, and Nelson (1995), reported that MVAs are the most frequently experienced trauma for American males (25% lifetime), and the second most frequently experienced trauma for females (13.8%). Norris (1992) found that MVAs were the leading cause of PTSD in the general population. As these studies illustrate, MVAs are prevalent, traumatic experiences in the United States.

While there has been an growing literature dealing with psychological consequences of MVAs (Blanchard & Hickling, 1997), to date little has appeared in that literature dealing with the treatment of PTSD following MVAs. The earliest mention of psychological consequences of MVAs focused upon a post-traumatic phobic response related to driving rather than to PTSD. The earlier cases, in fact, may have been PTSD but were undiagnosed due to the diagnostic formulations of that era. It has only been since 1980, with the publication of the *Diagnostic and Statistical Manual of Mental Disorders,* 3rd edition (DSM-III; American Psychiatric Association), that codification for the disorder of PTSD became uniform and that direct evaluation of PTSD treatments has become possible. However, due to the importance of the earlier work, it will be briefly summarized, before the PTSD treatment of MVA victims is reviewed.

THE TREATMENT OF ACCIDENT PHOBIA

The earliest MVA-related treatment literature we have been able to find has been that of Wolpe (1962) and Kraft and Al-Issa (1965). Both report on the use of systematic desensitization in the treatment of MVA-related phobias. Wolpe (1962) treated a woman who had been struck by a truck while driving through an intersection. The 39-year-old woman was rendered unconscious and transported to the hospital by ambulance. Upon the return home from the hospital following her hospital stay, she became "unaccountably frightened." She reported heightened anxiety when driving, which worsened when a car approached on either side. She had prior traumatic experiences, including a MVA at age 10 and the death of her fiancé, a pilot, who was killed during World War-II. Treatment was based on conditioning theories as applied to anxiety and phobic avoidance. More than 57 desensitization sessions were performed. In addition, treatment included hypnosis and imaginal desensitization. She was able to return to driving in normal traffic situations and was completely at ease despite near misses, without any long-lasting emotional consequence.

Kraft and Il-Issa (1965) treated a 37-year-old male who had two road accidents, which occurred while he was painting white lines on the road. The patient had a prior history of medical discharge from the army. Kraft and Il-Issa used three sessions of hypnotherapy, 22 sessions of desensitization (1½ hours each) and 10 follow-up sessions. Six months after treatment the patient was reported to be free of all symptoms. It was noted by the authors that the patient's symptoms had remitted prior to a legal settlement, lowering any consideration of secondary gain.

More recently, Quirk (1985) has also shown a reduction in MVA-related anxiety using similar techniques.

Taylor and Koch (1995) have pointed out that the systematic desensitization and other methods of imaginal exposure have been effective for some aspects of the MVA treatment that cannot be reproduced by in vivo exposure. Recent studies have, in fact, utilized both imaginal exposure and in vivo exposure. For example, Blonstein (1988) treated an accident phobic individual over 33 sessions using 22 weeks of imaginal exposure followed by 11 weeks of graduated in vivo exposure. Several other case studies have used similar approaches including Horne (1993), Levine and Wolpe (1980) and Rovetto (1983). The latter two cases, in fact, used in vivo desensitization while in radio contact with the patient. Rovetto (1983) utilized telemonitoring of psychophysiological responsiveness as well as verbal reports from the subject in the vehicle.

TREATMENT OF MVA-RELATED PTSD

McCaffrey and Fairbank (1985) utilized a broad spectrum assessment and treatment package for two individuals who had met DSM-III criteria for PTSD secondary to transportation accidents. One survivor's transportation accident was a helicopter crash, the second victim was a 20-year-old female who had been in four MVAs over a 14-month period of time. McCaffrey and Fairbank (1985) provided a treatment which consisted of three components: Relaxation training, flooding in imagination (implosive therapy to fearful stimulus), and self-directed in vivo exposure to the fear stimulus. At the end of treatment there was a reported drop in PTSD symptoms and a drop in skin conductance with exposure to fearful stimuli.

Kuch, Swinson, & Kirby (1985) assessed 30 (22 female, 8 male) MVA survivors, 12 of whom received treatment following a medical and legal evaluation. The 12 treatment subjects were provided four to eight hours of imaginal flooding, which included images of their accident and in vivo exposure to driving or being driven for no less than one and up to three hours per session for four sessions. Six of the 12 subjects were found to have marked improvement in symptoms, while four others improved their ability to drive following the provision of medication. Treatment subjects were also provided several hours of cognitively-oriented psychotherapy. Two subjects reportedly received no benefit from treatment and remained unable to drive. In a later paper, Kuch (1989) shared concerns about the occurrence of post-traumatic phobia, victimization by the system of survivors of MVAs, and the implications of chronic pain as it relates to the PTSD symptoms.

Studies by Muse (1986), McMillan (1991), and Horton (1993) have also reported anecdotal treatments of MVA-related PTSD. Horne (1993) reported on three cases, each of whom suffered psychological problems for at least six months after the MVA. Treatment included imaginal exposure to a hierarchy of car travel scenes, in vivo exposure, relaxation training, cognitive-behavioral therapy and conjoint sessions with significant others. Horne reported positive treatment results, although he cautioned that a considerable number of residual problems remained at the end of one year of treatment.

Lyons and Scotti (1995) reported on the use of a direct therapeutic exposure intervention and the value of adjunctive treatments of communication, anger control, marital and family therapy, and the importance of the therapeutic relationship. Lyons and Scotti, unfortunately reported that their case ended prematurely due to the subject's failure to report for treatment. Best and Ribbe (1995) described their approach to treatment of a 23-year-old male who had been in a serious MVA. Treatment involved a combination of relaxation training, cognitive interventions and behavioral techniques to address issues related to perceived life-threat, extended physical injury, reminders of the injury, and the role of therapist as an advocate for the patient. Unfortunately, they did not report any treatment outcomes for their illustrative case.

Brom, Kleber, and Hoffman (1993) have conducted the only controlled intervention study to date for MVA of the effectiveness of a psychological intervention designed to stimulate healthy coping behaviors following an MVA. Treatment included information, support for the victim and assistance with coping. Participants were assigned either to a control group or a group which utilized treatment over three sessions which could be extended to six sessions. Six months after the MVA, it was found that about half of the survivors continued to show moderate to severe symptoms of intrusion and avoidance. About 90% of the intervention group had indicated that they were content or very content with the intervention, but there appeared to be no significant difference in the degree of improvement on the Impact of Event Scale (IES) between the intervention group and the monitoring control group. Thus, the Brom et al. early intervention was no more effective than the passage of time.

In summary, the case study reports on a treatment of PTSD found in MVAs are, in general, very encouraging. Treatment, often follows a cognitive-behavioral model. Behavior treatments tend to utilize both imaginal and in vivo exposure techniques. These techniques have been reported for several decades. Cognitive models utilizing a variety of techniques that include thought stopping, cognitive reappraisal and cognitive reframing have been used to address issues related to mortality, the impact of pain or lingering physical injury, and driving phobia. It was based upon this backdrop of information that the Albany MVA Treatment Project was begun.

ALBANY MVA TREATMENT PROJECT:
TREATMENT STUDY 1

The initial effort at treatment at the Albany MVA Treatment Project arose from our experience conducting a National Institute of Mental Health (NIMH) funded research project investigating the psychological effects of motor vehicle accidents (Blanchard & Hickling, 1997). As part of the ethical responsibilities in the completion of that study, all MVA survivors who were found to have psychological difficulties were referred to a local treatment provider. The treatment, conducted by private psychologists, two of whom were associated with the MVA research project, offered a unique opportunity to measure the change in symptoms across time. Each intervention was individually tailored to the patient, as is typical in private practice, however, the overall treatment rationale for both treating psychologists was largely cognitive-behavioral. This similarity in treatment approach allowed for a comparison of treatment commonalties and differences. A more comprehensive description of this study can be found in Mitchell's (1997) recent text (Hickling et al., 1997).

Participants in the first study were two males and 10 females. Payment for psychological treatment was provided through "no fault" insurance. Prior to referral for treatment, all participants, as part of the MVA assessment research project, had undergone a comprehensive evaluation by one of the four experienced doctoral level psychologists familiar with PTSD assessments. PTSD was diagnosed utilizing criteria outlined in DSM-III-R (1987) and based upon the Clinician-Administered PTSD Scale (CAPS) (Blake et al., 1990). A thorough description of all outcome measures may be found elsewhere (Hickling, Loos, Blanchard, & Taylor, 1996).

All 12 participants received some type of exposure-based treatment, either in office imaginal exposure or graded in vivo exposure, in addition to relaxation training. Treatment for driving-related reluctance or phobia secondary to the MVA, or both, was provided to 11 of the 12 participants. Cognitive techniques were utilized with each participant and included thought stopping, guided self-dialogue, confrontation with the feared situation and management of anxiety, cognitive restructuring, and modeling and role playing for anxiety provoking situations. Treatment length varied considerably. This was consistent with the work of Burstein (1986) who had found that while a large number of MVA survivors improved in less than three months; a large number of individuals also required treatment of greater than one year. Ten of the twelve patients showed improvement in their CAPS scores across the 12-month period of time and showed corresponding improvements on psychological test measures.

TREATMENT RATIONALE

Based upon our experience with the MVA assessment study and the initial efforts of treatment, we have developed an understanding of the symptom clusters somewhat different than that found in DSM-IV (APA, 1994): This conceptualization has been useful in the overall treatment of MVA victims with PTSD. First, we believe there are four symptom clusters of importance: (a) reexperiencing, (b) avoidance, (c) psychic numbing, and (d) hyperarousal. This conceptualization of symptom clusters is useful, as each of these symptom clusters is addressed by designated psychological treatments.

Reexperiencing is best approached by vicarious exposure and forced reexperiencing of the trauma coupled with education and cognitive therapy to help the patient interpret the event and its outcome. One focus of intervention has been to try to help patients understand that reexperiencing symptoms should be expected and are part of the normal reaction to any significant trauma. Secondly, vicarious exposure can then occur by having the patients, either verbally or in writing, confront their personalized descriptions of the MVA and their subsequent emotional reactions to that confrontation. The variety of MVA experiences (e.g., lying in a car, trapped overnight; being extricated using the "jaws-of-life," seeing a second vehicle bearing down on them, or sliding out of control on icy surfaces) are unique to each person and consistent with the need for individualized exposure for patient improvement. The patient is helped to confront as many aspects of the cognitive network for the difficult memories as possible within a supportive therapeutic environment.

Avoidance symptoms can be approached through education, graded exposure homework, applied relaxation, and cognitive techniques. We have utilized the Two-Factor Learning Theory to explore the development of PTSD in MVA survivors (Keane, Zimering, & Caddell, 1985; Mowrer, 1947).

As Litz (1992) has pointed out, *psychic numbing and estrangement* are the least well-studied and understood cluster of symptoms making up PTSD. We have tended to view this cluster of symptoms (inability to recall important aspects of the MVA, diminished interest or participation in significant activities, detachment or estrangement from others, restricted range of affect, and a sense of foreshortened future) as closely resembling depression (feeling sad or empty, having decreased concentration, irritability, diminished interest or pleasure in all or most activities, feelings of worthlessness, recurrent thoughts of death, and symptoms causing distress or impairment in social or occupational functioning). We have subsequently utilized specific behavioral techniques (PES) and cognitive techniques to address the schema or irrational beliefs, or both, thought to contribute to this symptom cluster.

The impact on driving in our culture has also been found to be of great importance. Many people will endure driving that's necessary in their daily life, but will avoid any driving which may be viewed as optional or less than a dire necessity.

With regard to hyperarousal, relaxation has been shown to be an effective technique in helping counter symptoms of arousal in a war veteran population (Hickling, Sison, & Vanderploeg, 1986). We have found relaxation to be valuable to the MVA population.

Based upon our initial work, we believed the patients with MVA-related PTSD typically present with some combination of these four symptom clusters. Treatment should consequently include procedures to address all four of the symptom clusters, with a relative emphasis on those symptoms thought most important for each patient's idiosyncratic symptom presentation.

TREATMENT STUDY 2

Based upon the success of a nonsystematic initial intervention, a treatment manual for MVA victims with PTSD was designed. The treatment manual describes 9 to 12 sessions designed to address the symptoms of each individual patient while maintaining the clinical judgment of experienced clinicians.

Participants were recruited from advertisements in local newspapers and physician referrals. There were approximately 110 telephone inquiries, with 64 MVA survivors being screened for possible PTSD or subsyndromal PTSD symptoms by use of the PTSD Checklist (Weathers, Litz, Herman, Huska, & Keane, 1993). From the telephone interviews, 25 MVA survivors were seen for further evaluation, with 21 keeping their appointment for the comprehensive assessment. Out of that group of subjects, 12 were seen for treatment using the manual-based intervention. Two dropped out of treatment. Treatment was provided at no cost. Participants who completed treatment were reassessed at the end of treatment by independent evaluators.

Participants

Participants for this study were 10 MVA survivors (9 female, 1 male) with a mean age of 45.6 years. All were survivors of MVAs that had occurred at least six months prior to the time of the initial evaluation and had sought medical attention for injuries related to the MVA within 72 hours of their accidents. The rationale for treating survivors who had symptoms for at least six months came from the results of an earlier study which showed the PTSD symptoms were fairly stable after six months (Blanchard et al., 1995). In our initial assessment study, 50% of those who had met criteria for PTSD shortly after the MVA no longer did so by six months. Our rationale was that, if MVA survivors showed symptoms after a six-month period of time, they were less likely to show improvement spontaneously from that point on. Consequently, any change in our criterion measures would be more likely to reflect treatment effects rather than any spontaneous improvement.

Evaluation Methods

The diagnosis for PTSD was established through use of the CAPS (Blake et al., 1990). All interviews were taped and reviewed. MVA survivors were diagnosed as having PTSD based upon DSM-IV criteria (APA, 1994). Participants were also asked to complete the Beck Depression Inventory (BDI; Beck, Ward, Mendelson, Mock, & Erbaugh, 1961), State-Trait Anxiety Inventory (STAI; Spielberger, Gorsuch, & Lushene, 1970). To obtain self-report measures of PTSD symptoms, the Impact of Event Scale (IES; Horowitz, Wilmer, & Alvarez, 1979) and the Post-Traumatic Checklist (PCL; Weathers et al., 1993) were used.

Subjects also underwent a locally-constructed interview on their MVA and their reaction to their MVA. Psychosocial functioning for each MVA victim was determined through the use of the LIFE-Base Interview (Keller et al., 1987).

Follow-up evaluations were completed at the conclusion of treatment and at a three-month posttreatment follow-up session by independent evaluators (advanced doctoral students in clinical psychology).

Intervention was based on a symptom-focused psychological treatment designed to address MVA-related PTSD and subsyndromal PTSD-related symptoms. An outline of session-by-session treatment topics from our revised manual can be found in Table 6.1. A more thorough description of this study may be found elsewhere (Hickling & Blanchard, 1997).

Treatment results were positive for all 10 MVA victims. CAPS scores across treatment by the three assessments yield a main effect ($F(2,7) = 10.4$, $p = .008$, Pillais) but there is no main effect for therapist or interaction of therapist by assessment. There was a significant drop in CAPS score from pretreatment to posttreatment but no further improvement from posttreatment to follow-up. Five of the eight MVA victims who had started with full PTSD were at a non-PTSD level by the end of treatment. The remaining three MVA survivors had decreased symptoms sufficient to be diagnosed as subsyndromal PTSD. By the three-month follow-up, two of these three survivors improved further to no longer fit the PTSD diagnosis. Scores on the psychological tests, including the measures of psychosocial functioning were also found to improve significantly.

TABLE 6.1. Manualized Treatment Protocol for Motor Vehicle Accident-Related PTSD

Major Theme/Content for Session	Assignment/Homework for Next Session
Session 1: Review MVA description; review PTSD Rationale & Treatment Rationale; introduce 16 muscle group relaxation; provide tape of 16 muscle group relaxation.	Patient to write out complete MVA description; practice and rate success of relaxation exercises.
Session 2: Complete/elaborate MVA description; have patient read MVA description aloud; discuss role of avoidance; repeat 16 muscle group relaxation.	Ask if significant other can join next time; continue with daily reading of MVA description; continue with twice daily practice of 16 muscle group relaxation.
Session 3: Review MVA description aloud; discuss homework; introduce self-coping statements; begin avoidance hierarchy; meet with significant other; introduce 8-muscle group relaxation; provide audio tape of 8-muscle group relaxation.	Daily review of description of MVA: begin application of self-coping statements; practice 8-muscle group relaxation exercises; continue to develop avoidance hierarchy.
Session 4: Reading exposure to MVA; discuss homework; review hierarchy; introduce cognitive reappraisal; introduce 4-muscle group relaxation.	Continue with daily review of MVA description; encourage exposure to driving/avoidance hierarchy; continue with use of self-coping statements & cognitive reappraisal of anxiety provoking events; to practice with either 8 or 4 muscle group relaxation exercises.
Session 5: Reading exposure to MVA description adding in imaginal exposure to situations that are feared but rarely occurring from driving hierarchy; discuss homework; review avoidance hierarchy and discuss any difficulties, while emphasizing coping self-statements and cognitive restructuring; introduce relaxation by recall.	Continue with daily reading of MVA description; daily practice with relaxation by recall; continued exposure to avoidance hierarchy.
Session 6: Reading exposure to MVA (if patient is no longer demonstrating reactivity to MVA reading, reduce patient's exposure to once daily); introduce cue-controlled relaxation; review hierarchy, discuss cognitive strategies used.	Continue with reading exposure to MVA; daily practice with cue-controlled relaxation training; continued exposure to avoidance hierarchy, utilizing cognitive reappraisal and self-talk techniques.

Table 6.1 continues on page 110.

TABLE 6.1. *Continued*

Major Theme/Content for Session	Assignment/Homework for Next Session
Session 7: Review cognitive/behavioral treatment to date and encourage continued home practice; discuss homework; begin discussion of patient symptoms/reactions reviewed in the initial session, discuss current feelings and explore possible signs of depression; discuss themes of existential issues, social isolation, lack of positive events, pleasant events scheduling (PES), and anger management.	Continue with reading exposure adjusted as patient response; continued exposure to avoidance hierarchy with utilization of cognitive techniques; daily application of pleasant events scheduling; other homework assignments as applicable from themes introduced in Session 7.
Session 8: Review driving and behavioral avoidance hierarchy; review pleasant events scheduling and difficulties; check on social activity and social involvement; explore possible cognitive schema related to depression and apply cognitive restructuring; explore possible avoidance of strong affect and develop methods to increase exposure to those affect.	Reading of MVA description can be discontinued if no reaction continues at this time; suggest occasional (once or twice week) return to full 16-muscle group relaxation exercise; continue with PES; continue with exposure/imaginal homework as appropriate.
Session 9: Same as Session 8.	Same as Session 8.
Session 10: Final Visit; Review Symptoms from Session 1, comparing changes or lack of progress; encourage continued home practice as appropriate; review treatment (exposure, cognitive techniques, etc.); terminate treatment, or set goals for continued treatment.	Completion of standardized assessment procedures to allow measurement of change across treatment.

Overall, the CAPS score changes strongly suggest that the manualized-based treatment protocol was effective in the reduction of symptoms of PTSD in survivors of MVAs. These results also strongly suggest that the symptom improvements can be obtained in a short period of time and that the gains are durable over time. The study was uncontrolled and thus has many limitations, including the possibility that improvement would have occurred over time anyway. However, based upon a naturalistic follow-up of MVA survivors, only 5% of those who have PTSD at six months fully remitted by 12 months, while another 5% showed some partial improvements spontaneously (Blanchard et al., 1995). Consequently, this pilot investigation suggests significantly greater improvement than would be expected without an effective treatment being in place.

We have recently begun a formal, controlled investigation of the most recent revision of the treatment manual.

SUGGESTIONS FOR PSYCHOLOGICAL TREATMENT, INCLUDING GROUP APPLICATION

Based upon our work to date, we believe there are several important components of individual psychological intervention that could be applied to group intervention for MVA victims with PTSD. These components are as follows:

1 *Evaluation.* It is important that the patient understand the diagnosis and the symptoms that comprise the diagnosis. The logic and development of the diagnosis allow the patient and psychologist to begin with a shared place of intervention. Rapport-building is also established through the evaluation process, and, in practice, this is an invaluable beginning from which an individualized treatment plan may be formulated. An obvious time for this to occur is during the interview for entry into a group. The use of screening instruments to aid in diagnosis may help both the clinician and patient understand the particular areas of problems to be addressed in treatment prior to the first treatment session.

2 *Education.* An important part of the psychological intervention is to provide information regarding reactions to trauma and reassurance that an individual is not *going crazy.* Our conceptualization of PTSD and the symptom clusters may be addressed in psychological treatments and provide a rationale by which the therapist and the patient can agree to a course of improvement. We let individuals know that as many as 40% of MVA survivors who seek medical treatment after a MVA, may have PTSD or a milder form of it, shortly after their trauma. Education can easily be provided in a group format, and it is readily adaptable to groups of different composition (e.g. family members as well as victims) and size.

3 *Relaxation training.* We found that progressive relaxation training (Bernstein & Borkovec, 1973) or shorter versions of relaxation provide an invaluable tool for the patient. He or she gains a skill to apply to the MVA-related anxiety and to use during subsequent exposure-based interventions. Relaxation training can be readily adapted to a group format.

4 *Exposure.* Whether delivered via imaginal exposure or graded in vivo desensitization, we believe that exposure is an essential part of psychological intervention. We often start this exposure by having patients write the description of their MVA and then, over the course of treatment, have them read that description to themselves several times each day. In addition to the exposure that occurs within the session, this homework provides a consistent and, we believe, invaluable exposure to the stimulus which can trigger their PTSD symptoms.

Research evidence and our own experience suggest that exposure is critical for reducing PTSD symptoms. The written description technique could be modified for the group context and employed as a homework assignment, to be followed up in subsequent sessions. Difficulties that arise in completion of the task could be addressed, and shared by group members.

5 *Cognitive therapy.* Patients are instructed in coping statements (Meichenbaum, 1985), and a stress inoculation training method for preparing for situations in dealing with stressful situations, is rapidly offered. This therapy naturally leads into the cognitive reappraisal and ABC model for intervention with irrational thoughts (e.g., Ellis, 1962), which we have found to be useful for helping patients deal with the distortions and cognitions which lead to anxiety and avoidance. The use of cognitive educational techniques is certainly applicable to a group format, and the provision of a group may in many ways facilitate the procedure by allowing the MVA survivors to hear similar cognitive distortions and adaptations in others.

6 *Spouse.* Involvement of spouses has proven to be an invaluable component of many patients' treatment. Partners play a large, and often essential, role in the MVA survivor's life. By trying to be helpful, they often unwittingly enable the survivors to continue the avoidance of the driving- or MVA-related reactions. Spouses often do not understand, and may even be hostile toward, the changes that have occurred in their partners. Consequently, the provision of education, an explanation of the disorder, and a rationale for treatment can be of great benefit. Spouses are often included in driving exposure treatment and can provide invaluable support in treatment. The use of the spouse within and outside the group holds considerable promise for aiding treatment efforts. In fact, group therapy might be a powerful factor in helping the victims whose spouses publicly share their perceptions and, at times, skepticism or lack of understanding about the changes that have occurred to their significant other.

7 *Driving.* One area of impact almost universally found among MVA survivors in our research and clinical experience has been the adverse effect on driving. Many individuals will avoid the site of their MVA while others may cease all driving. The impact of the MVA on driving can vary considerably. A behavioral intervention for driving may be introduced with an exposure-based intervention which utilizes the spouse or the patient solely. Driving is seen by many to hold an element of risk. This belief is dealt with utilizing cognitive techniques, as well as reassurance of the survivor's driving skills which the patient will rely upon in treatment and future driving efforts. The application to group appears straight forward, and could follow guidelines found in phobia treatment approaches which use a group format.

8 *Anger control.* Patients often experience a great deal of anger as a result of the changes they have been forced to undergo, changes that are often no fault of their own. They may also be angry at the legal system, which limits their capability to return to work or obtain disability benefits. They are often placed in adversarial positions, rather than being seen as victims trying to regain important aspects of their lives. Methods of dealing with anger include behavioral and cognitive techniques (Novaco, 1975), consistent with treatment addressing PTSD symptoms. Anger management training also holds promise for group application.

9 *Pleasant events scheduling (PES).* Consistent with our conceptualization of psychic numbing, pleasant events scheduling (Lewinsohn & Libet, 1972) has been found as a useful intervention for many of the MVA survivors. Pleasant events scheduling is a technique developed from the application of social learning theory for the treatment of depression. As Lewinsohn, Antonuccio, Steinmetz, and Teri (1984) point out, the guiding assumption for pleasant events scheduling is that the restoration of an adequate schedule of positive reinforcement is critical in the amelioration of dysphoria. This principle, then, guides treatment to alter the frequency, quality, and range of the patient's activities and social interactions. The avoidance of activities, the diminished interest or participation in activities, the restricted range of affect, difficulty concentrating, irritability, and sense of foreshortened future all parallel feelings found in depressed individuals. While only clinical experience led to the initial trial of these techniques, the clinical data is now being assembled that supports this intervention. PES also helps to increase socialization and sociability; in general, PES is a useful adjunctive intervention for a majority of survivors. PES is also helpful for patients who present with comorbid depression.

10 *Existential issues.* One common theme found in MVA survivors has been a fear of death and graphic imagery of one's mortality. We have found it useful to address these concerns in the therapeutic relationship, and to allow them to be explored in a safe and supportive environment. On many occasions the impact of near death raises questions about spirituality and religion. Survivors often seek reasons as to why the MVA occurred and wonder about how to draw meaning from the accident within their life. One's spiritual beliefs are often tested, and openly discussing those beliefs in a therapeutic environment is often of great benefit. The use of a group where these issues can be shared also holds significant potential.

We believe very strongly in the provision of an individually-based treatment intervention. However, based upon our work to date, a manualized-based intervention assures that what appear to be the most potent components of treatment are provided. It is also important to understand that trauma prior to the MVA is at times critical in the shaping of PTSD following MVAs, and should also be addressed within the course of psychotherapeutic intervention.

GROUP THERAPY WITH MVA SURVIVORS

Our work to date has solely focused on the provision of psychotherapeutic interventions with individuals. Our literature search has not found any interventions for groups of MVA survivors. We believe that the psychological intervention, however, could very easily be addressed within a group setting. The themes found within the individual sessions of the treatment manual could easily be tailored to a group model, as suggested above. This tailoring could also include the provision of spouses, behavioral interventions for driving, and exposure to feared situations. The supportive aspects of group therapy and the therapeutic benefits have been realized in many other trauma-related populations. It is reasonable to assume that these same benefits can be obtained for MVA trauma survivors.

Relaxation and cognitive techniques can be readily delivered in group settings, and group application may prove to be one of the most cost-effective and time-efficient methods for delivering these psychological interventions. At this point, however, and given the absence of data at this time, we can only speculate about the potential benefits. Research is needed to support these seemingly logical extensions from the literature on the treatment of individuals.

The time and effort it takes to develop a therapy group can be considerable. However, it is not unlikely that opportunities for group treatment of PTSD following a MVA will emerge and will be developed in the foreseeable future. This is thought to be true for several reasons. First, those individuals who have not improved after several months, in all likelihood, will still require psychological intervention. Thus, it may be possible to gather enough individuals to provide group therapy with a reasonable effort. A second scenario for group intervention may be that of a large scale transportation disaster, such as a bus or multiple car accident. It is hoped that, for such tragedies, treatment guidelines suggested from the current literature will aide the practitioners helping MVA survivors.

REFERENCES

American Psychiatric Association. (1980). *Diagnostic and statistical manual of mental disorders* (3rd ed.). Washington, DC: Author.

American Psychiatric Association. (1994). *Diagnostic and statistical manual of mental disorders* (4th ed.). Washington, DC: Author.

Beck, A. T., Ward, C. H., Mendelson, M., Mock, J., & Erbaugh, J. (1961). An inventory for measuring depression. *Archives of General Psychiatry, 5,* 561–571.

Bernstein, D. A., & Borkovec, T. D. (1973). *Progressive relaxation training: A manual for the helping professions.* Champaign, IL: Research Press.

Best, C. L., & Ribbe, D. P. (1995). Accidental injury: Approaches to assessment and treatment. In J. R. Freedy & S. E. Hobfoil (Eds.), *Traumatic stress: From theory to practice.* New York: Plenum Press.

Blake, D., Weathers, F., Nagy, L., Kaloupek, D., Klauminzer, G., Charney, D., & Keane, T. (1990). *Clinician-administered PTSD scale (CAPS).* Boston: National Center for Post-Traumatic Stress Disorder, Behavioral Science Division.

Blanchard, E. B., & Hickling, E. J. (In press). *After the crash: Psychological assessment and treatment of survivors of motor vehicle accidents.* Washington, DC: American Psychological Association.

Blanchard, E. B., Hickling, E. J., Vollmer, A. J., Loos, W. R., Buckley, T. C., & Jaccard, J. (1995). Short–term follow-up of post-traumatic stress symptoms in motor vehicle accident victims. *Behaviour Research and Therapy, 33,* 369–377.

Blonstein, C. H. (1988). Treatment of automobile driving phobia through imaginal and in vivo exposure plus response prevention. *The Behavior Therapist, 11,* 70–86.

Brom, D., Kleber, R. J., & Hoffman, M. C. (1993). Victims of traffic accidents: Incidence and prevention of post-traumatic stress disorder. *Journal of Clinical Psychology, 49,* 131–140.

Burstein, A. (1986). Treatment length in post-traumatic stress disorder. *Psychosomatics, 27,* 632–637.

Ellis, A. (1962). *Reason and emotion in psychotherapy.* New York: Lyle Stuart.

Hickling, E. J., & Blanchard, E. B. (1997). The private practice psychologist and manual-based treatment: A case study in the treatment of post-traumatic stress disorder secondary to motor vehicle accidents. *Behaviour Research and Therapy, 35,* 191–203.

Hickling, E. J., Blanchard, E. B., Schwarz, S. P., & Silverman, D. J. (1992). Headaches and motor vehicle accidents: Results of psychological treatment of post-traumatic headache. *Headache Quarterly, 30,* 285–289.

Hickling, E. J., Loos, W. R., Blanchard, E. B., & Taylor, A. E. (1996). Treatment of post-traumatic stress disorder (PTSD) after road accidents. In M. Mitchell (Ed.), *Road accidents: The social and psychological impact of any everyday trauma.* London: Routledge.

Hickling, E. J., Sison, G.F.P., & Vanderploeg, K. D. (1986). The treatment of post-traumatic stress disorder with biofeedback and relaxation training. *Biofeedback and Self-Regulation, 11,* 125–134.

Horne, D. J. (1993). Traumatic stress reactions to motor vehicle accidents. In J. P. Wilson & B. Raphael (Eds.), *International handbook of traumatic stress syndromes* (pp. 499–506). New York: Plenum Press.

Horowitz, M. J., Wilmer, N., & Alvarez, N. (1979). Impact of event scale: A measure of subjective stress. *Psychosomatic Medicine, 41,* 209–218.

Horton, A. M. (1993). Post-traumatic stress disorder and mild head trauma: Follow-up of a case study. *Perceptual and Motor Skills, 76,* 243–246.

Keane, T. M., Zimering, R. T., & Caddell, J. M. (1985). A behavioral formulation of post-traumatic stress disorder. *The Behavior Therapist, 8,* 9–12.

Keller, M. B., Lavori, P. W., Friedman, B., Nielsen, E., Endicott, J., McDonald-Scott, P., & Andreasen, N. C. (1987). A longitudinal interval follow-up evaluation: A comprehensive method for assessing outcome and prospective longitudinal studies. *Archives of General Psychiatry, 44,* 540–548.

Kraft, T., & Al-Issa, I. (1965). The application of learning theory to the treatment of traffic phobia. *British Journal of Psychiatry, 111,* 277–279.

Kuch, K. (1987). Treatment of PTSD following automobile accidents. *The Behavior Therapist, 10,* 224–242.

Kuch, K. (1989). Treatment of post-traumatic phobias and PTSD after car accidents. In P. A. Keller & S. R. Hayman (Eds.), *Innovations in clinical practice: A source book* (vol. 8, pp. 263–271). Sarasota, FL: Professional Resource Exchange.

Kuch, K., Swinson, R. P., & Kirby, M. (1985). Post-traumatic stress disorder after car accidents. *Canadian Journal of Psychiatry, 30,* 426–427.

Levine, B. A., & Wolpe, J. (1980). *In vivo* desensitization of a severe driving phobia through radio contact. *Journal of Behavior Therapy and Experiment Psychiatry, 11,* 281–282.

Lewinsohn, P. M., Antonuccio, D., Steinmetz, J., & Teri, L. (1984). *The coping with depression course: A psychoeducational intervention for unipolar depression.* Eugene, OR: Castalia.

Lewinsohn, P. M., & Libet, J. (1972). Pleasant events activity schedule and depression. *Journal of Abnormal Psychology, 79,* 291–295.

Litz, B. T. (1992). Emotional numbing in combat-related post-traumatic stress disorder: A clinical review and reformulation. *Clinical Psychology Review, 12,* 417–432.

Lyons, J. A., & Scotti, J. R. (1995). Behavioral treatment of a motor vehicle accident survivor: An illustrative case of direct therapist exposure. *Cognitive and Behavioral Practice, 2,* 343–364.

McCaffrey, R. J., & Fairbank, J. A. (1985). Behavioral assessment and treatment of accident-related post-traumatic stress disorder: Two case studies. *Behavior Therapy, 16,* 406–416.

McMillan, T. M. (1991). Post-traumatic stress disorder and severe head injury. *British Journal of Psychiatry, 159,* 431–433.

Meichenbaum, D. (1985). *Stress inoculation training.* New York: Pergamon Press.

Mitchell, M. (1997). *The aftermath of road accidents.* London: Routledge.

Mowrer, O. H. (1947). On the dual nature of learning: The reinterpretation of "conditioning" and "problem solving." *Harvard Educational Review, 17,* 102–148.

Muse, M. (1986). Stress-related post-traumatic chronic pain syndrome: Behavioral approach to treatment. *Pain, 25,* 389–394.

Novaco, R. W. (1975). *Anger control.* Lexington, MA: Lexington Press.

Quirk, D. A. (1985). Motor vehicle accidents and post-traumatic anxiety conditioning. *The Ontario Psychologist, 17,* 11–18.

Rovetto, F. M. (1983). *In vivo* desensitization of a severe driving phobia through radio contact with telemonitoring of neurophysiological reactors. *Journal of Behavior Therapy and Experimental Psychiatry, 14,* 49–54.

Spielberger, C. D., Gorsuch, R. L., & Lushene, R. E. (1970). *STAI manual for the state-trait anxiety inventory.* Palo Alto, CA: Consulting Psychologists Press.

Taylor, S., & Koch, W. T. (1995). Anxiety disorders due to motor vehicle accidents: Nature and treatment. *Clinical Psychology Review, 15,* 721–738.

Weathers, F. W., Litz, B. T., Herman, D. S., Huska, J. A., & Keane, T. M. (1993, October). *The PTSD checklist: Reliability, validity & diagnostic utility.* Paper presented at the annual meeting of the International Society for Traumatic Stress Studies, San Antonio, TX.

Wolpe, J. (1962). Isolation of a conditioning procedure as the crucial psychotherapeutic factor: A case study. *Journal of Nervous and Mental Disease, 134,* 316–329.

Wolpe, J. (1973). *The practice of behavior therapy* (2nd ed.). New York: Pergamon Press.

Chapter 7

Group Treatment of PTSD and Comorbid Alcohol Abuse

Andrew W. Meisler

Alcohol use disorders are a common and clinically challenging problem among individuals with post-traumatic stress disorder (PTSD). Prevalence estimates of alcohol abuse among trauma victims seeking treatment for PTSD have ranged as high as 75% (e.g., Keane, Gerardi, Lyons, & Wolfe, 1988). Often, these individuals suffer from comorbid anxiety or depressive disorders as well as other substance use disorders, further complicating evaluation and treatment. Yet, only recently have systematic approaches to treatment been developed for these dual disorders. Historically, individuals with PTSD and substance abuse problems were often caught between different treatment systems with different philosophies. Treatment for PTSD in traditional mental health settings was often insensitive to the critical role of alcohol abuse or, worse, was refused because of comorbid substance abuse. Patients would then be referred to substance abuse treatment settings, where the important interplay and overlap of PTSD symptoms and alcohol use was often overlooked. Fortunately, the last 10 to 15 years has seen significant growth in knowledge and clinical application with dually-diagnosed individuals (e.g., Drake & Noordsy, 1996). These approaches emphasize integrated treatment of the whole person, rather than partitioning treatment into separate psychiatric and substance abuse components which often lack continuity of care. It is this integrative approach, in conjunction with mounting experience in applying established substance abuse treatment modalities to individuals with PTSD, that forms the basis for this chapter.

The purpose of this chapter is to describe the principles and techniques of group therapy for individuals with PTSD and comorbid alcohol use disorders. The majority of these techniques share a common cognitive-behavioral basis, an approach justified by the available treatment literature to date in both substance abuse and PTSD. The reader should be aware at the outset, however, that the majority of techniques covered in this chapter are based on clinical data and experience and relatively little outcome data. Much of this material reflects an integration of material that, until recently, remained largely independent. For example, group treatment has long been the standard of care for patients with alcohol use disorders. Group therapy has also gained prominence in the treatment of PTSD—as this volume attests—though individual approaches still play an important role. The principles and techniques described here reflect a rationally and empirically derived method for integrating these approaches in treating dually-diagnosed individuals. Moreover, this chapter is not a treatment manual that provides detailed instruction on how to deliver treatment. The chapter does, however, provide an overview of concepts and methods sufficient to familiarize the skilled clinician with the essential ingredients of treatment.

The chapter begins with a brief overview of empirical research on PTSD and alcohol comorbidity, including available data on group treatment outcome with this population. The chapter then outlines the fundamental principles and techniques of group therapy, including therapeutic rationale, treatment components, client selection, and troubleshooting.

EMPIRICAL RESEARCH IN PTSD/ALCOHOL ABUSE COMORBIDITY

Both epidemiologic and clinical studies have consistently documented a high prevalence of alcohol abuse in patients seeking treatment for PTSD. For example, in their oft-cited paper, Keane et al. (1988) summarized results of previous studies as well as their own data by suggesting that 60% to 80% of treatment-seeking Vietnam veterans with PTSD also met criteria for current alcohol or drug abuse, or both. More recently, Fontana, Rosenheck, Spencer, and Gray (1995) reported that 44% of veterans seeking outpatient treatment in VA specialized PTSD programs met criteria for alcohol abuse/dependence. Several studies of civilian trauma (e.g., sexual abuse) in treatment-seeking samples also suggest an increased prevalence of alcohol abuse, although these data are less consistent and the prevalence estimates are lower than in veteran samples. Conversely, both clinical and epidemiologic studies of substance abusers have demonstrated a significantly increased risk for both trauma and PTSD (e.g., Cottler, Compton, Mager, Spitznagel, & Ianca, 1992; Fullilove et al., 1993). Thus, just as trauma and PTSD may predispose to substance abuse, the reverse may also be true (for an excellent review of empirical research on PTSD/alcohol comorbidity, see Stewart, 1996).

These high comorbidity rates, in conjunction with the clinical challenge of working with these clients, have led many investigators to speculate about mechanisms of comorbidity. This literature, though limited in scope, has emphasized the role of PTSD symptoms and trauma-related variables in predicting alcohol use.

Abueg and Fairbank (1992) have referred to this as the "interaction argument." Many authors have invoked the concept of self-medication (Khantzian, 1985) as a model for understanding alcohol use in patients with PTSD. This notion is consistent with research on the tension reducing or stress dampening effects of alcohol on anxiety and stress reactivity (e.g., Levenson, Sher, Grossman, Newman, & Newlin, 1980), as well as with other literature on alcohol's effects on cognitive function (see Meisler, 1996a; Stewart, 1996).

A number of studies have yielded data which bear either directly or indirectly on the self-medication hypothesis. Green, Lindy, Grace, and Gleser (1989) found that, among Vietnam combat veterans, exposure to grotesque death (e.g., mutilation) or graves registration, or both, was predictive of alcohol abuse, although the presence of a prewar psychiatric condition also contributed significantly and independently to alcohol abuse comorbidity. In one of the best studies to date, McFall, McKay, and Donovan (1992) examined substance abuse patterns in a sample of 108 combat veterans and 151 noncombat controls. Alcohol and drug abuse was associated with both PTSD severity and combat-related variables. Interestingly, specific PTSD symptom patterns were predictive of substance use patterns; elevated arousal symptoms were associated with alcohol problems, whereas avoidance/numbing was associated with drug abuse. In contrast, epidemiologic data from combat veterans suggested that, although combat exposure was predictive of subsequent substance abuse, PTSD was not (Reifman & Windle, 1996).

An alternative conceptualization is that stress and other trauma-related material may serve as conditioned stimuli or cues for alcohol use. In a recent study, Meisler (1996b) examined the effect of combat cues, noncombat stressful cues, and neutral cues on craving for alcohol in Vietnam veterans with PTSD and alcohol dependence. Consistent with predictions, combat cues elicited the greatest urge to drink, greater even than exposure to alcohol cues in the absence of a stressor. Although further data are needed to clarify the contribution of trauma and PTSD to alcohol abuse, from a clinical perspective the acknowledgment of these factors and the interaction of PTSD and substance use is vital to successful treatment.

As our research base on PTSD and alcohol comorbidity is still in its infancy, so too is the treatment outcome literature. However, several scientist-practitioners have been developing group treatment for this population and have just now begun to report preliminary data on treatment efficacy. For example, Padin-Rivera, Donovan, and McCormick (1996) have developed a 12-week treatment program for veterans with combat-related PTSD and substance use disorders. Although the program is multimodal and includes individual therapy, exercise, and other activities, the core treatment comprises group therapy including educational, skills building, and process components that address PTSD and substance use simultaneously. Initial outcome and preliminary six-month follow-up data based on CAPS scores are encouraging (Padin-Rivera, Donovan, & McCormick, 1996). Najavits, Weiss, and Liese (1996) describe a manualized 24-session cognitive-behavioral group therapy for women with PTSD and comorbid substance use disorders designed for use in outpatient settings. The treatment also includes education and skills training, with additional emphasis on cognitive restructuring and relationship/communication skills. Preliminary outcome data indicate reductions in both PTSD and substance use at posttreatment and three-month follow-up with good treatment retention and patient satisfaction (Najavits, Weiss, & Shaw, 1996). Further development and evaluation of such treatments is vital if we are to expand our knowledge base and enhance treatment efficacy with this population.

PRINCIPLES AND TECHNIQUES

Therapeutic Rationale

The rationale for the group therapy outlined here comes from several sources. First, group therapy has several advantages over other treatment modalities. For the purpose of education, a group provides the most efficient way to communicate with clients. More importantly, a group of individuals with similar difficulties can provide a supportive and salutary environment for change. Often the knowledge that others share similar experiences and distress is helpful, as clients, prior to entering treatment, often feel isolated, guilty, and misunderstood. Thus the group context provides a safe environment for self-disclosure and reassurance.

Second, there is a strong rationale for treating both disorders together in one group rather than dividing treatments across traditional psychiatric and substance abuse domains. Integration of service improves continuity of care and contributes to clients' perceptions that they are being treated as whole persons. This argument and rationale for integrated treatment is strengthened by the fact that clients often have preconceived beliefs and expectancies about the relationship between PTSD and alcohol abuse. For example, clients often describe their alcohol use as an effort to manage reexperiencing and arousal symptoms of PTSD. Often, these attributions become firmly embedded in a cognitive schema for understanding and explaining their difficulties. Whether these explanations are ultimately true or not, they represent an important part of the client's view of his or her illness, and must be taken into account in treatment. One difficulty often encountered in work with the dually-diagnosed is that psychoeducation about the interaction of PTSD and alcohol use can actually be construed by patients as reinforcing the view that PTSD causes substance abuse, that they are not responsible for change, and that they can only stop drinking when the PTSD is treated or cured. It is therefore imperative for the therapist to emphasize that knowledge and awareness of PTSD/alcohol interactions enhance the patient's ability to manage their disorders more effectively, but do not relieve them of responsibility for change.

The content of group sessions is guided by the observation that PTSD and alcohol dependence do share many common features. First, reexperiencing symptoms, the hallmark of PTSD, are also present—albeit in a slightly different way—in substance use disorders. For example, there is considerable clinical evidence that intrusive thoughts in the form of craving play a strong role in relapse to alcohol (e.g., Marlatt & Gordon, 1985). Related intrusive phenomena include spending considerable time and effort planning drinking, determining how to get a drink, and imagining the act of drinking. Studies in cocaine (Tunis, Dehuehi, & Hall, 1994) and nicotine (Salkovskis & Reynolds, 1994) addiction, that have conceptualized craving as an intrusive thought, have supported the merit of this conceptualization for understanding treatment outcome and relapse. Thus cognitive-behavioral therapy techniques aimed at managing attentional processes are relevant for both PTSD and alcohol dependence. Second, both disorders also share a critical arousal component. The hyperarousal symptoms of PTSD and their neurobiologic substrate have been well documented (see Orr, 1994; Charney, Deutch, Krystal, Southwick, & Davis, 1993). Similarly, research has demonstrated exaggerated arousal in response to alcohol cues in alcoholics (e.g., Cooney, Baker, Pomerleau, & Josephy, 1984; Monti et al., 1987) and a number of studies have linked alcohol to a reduction or *dampening* of the stress response (e.g., Levenson, Sher, Grossman, Newman, & Newlin, 1980). Thus arousal reducing strategies (e.g., anger management or relaxation) are important for both disorders. Third, both PTSD and alcohol dependence share a reliance on avoidant coping strategies. In chronic alcohol dependence and PTSD, more active and problem-focused coping skills atrophy. In some cases, avoidance—in conjunction with alcohol use—often becomes the sole coping strategy. Hence, treatments designed to enhance social problem-solving as well as emotion management are critical for successful treatment.

Client Selection Considerations

There are a variety of client characteristics that impact on treatment. Although few client factors will necessarily preclude participation in treatment, there are a number of considerations that can influence the course and focus of treatment as well as prognosis. Careful assessment of these client factors using both structured interview and paper-and-pencil measures is essential prior to commencing group treatment.

Type of trauma is an obvious consideration in client selection. The treatment outlined in this chapter is based largely on experience with Vietnam combat veterans. However, the techniques are not specific to a particular trauma type. The emphasis here is on symptom profiles in PTSD and alcohol dependence, which can then be customized to suit the needs of the population. It is generally accepted clinically that homogeneous groups foster rapport and facilitate the group therapy process. Patients with similar trauma histories feel more comfortable discussing trauma-related material, and can provide support to one another that may otherwise be unavailable in a more heterogeneous group. However, just as clients with different addictions can benefit from mixed groups that emphasize commonalities across addictions, so too can PTSD clients with varied backgrounds. Ultimately, selection of clients based on trauma history will depend on the therapist's interest, the clinical demand, and the setting in which the work is done.

Clinicians are often reluctant to treat clients with a history of severe and refractory alcohol dependence or comorbid illicit drug use, or both. Generally, these clients are believed to adhere more poorly to treatment and have higher drop-out and relapse rates. We have found, however, that clients who are ready for change, regardless of history, respond well to the treatment components presented here. In this context it is useful to apply the concept of stages of change (cf. Prochaska & DiClemente, 1982). In this model, readiness for change is viewed as a fluid and changing factor in treatment rather than as a motivational concept or as an enduring part of the person's character. Research on stages of change in alcohol abuse has generally supported four stages: precontemplation, contemplation, action, and maintenance. Regardless of history, clients at the contemplation/action stages are generally ready for the treatment program presented here. Motivational components described below are particularly useful for clients in earlier stages of readiness for change.

One of the most pressing debates and perhaps the most difficult decision to make clinically is whether or not to begin treatment while a client is still actively drinking. Some have argued that substance use must be in remission prior to initiating treatment for PTSD. In fact, active substance use has often been listed as an exclusion for exposure-based PTSD treatment, citing risk of substance abuse exacerbation caused by exposure-induced anxiety and arousal. In contrast, two clinical reports have suggested that such treatment may actually lead to decreased drinking in patients with active alcohol problems (e.g., Keane & Kaloupek, 1982; Lacousiere, Godfrey, & Rubey, 1980). In general, clinicians must weigh the following factors in determining the appropriateness of initiating treatment with active drinkers:

- Has there been a recent exacerbation in frequency and/or severity of alcohol use relative to baseline? Have there been repeated unsuccessful attempts to stop in recent weeks?

- Does drinking serve as potent distractor which will interfere with commitment to treatment, group attendance, homework completion, etc.?

- Can the client set positive and realistic goals for change in drinking behavior and set these as a priority in the treatment?

- Will ongoing drinking have a negative impact on other group members' sobriety and their belief in the integrity of the treatment?

- Consideration of clinician's own model. Those who subscribe to a 12-step approach based on a disease model are less likely to tolerate moderate alcohol use, whereas those with a more behavioral background may view moderate intake as consistent with the notion of *harm reduction.*

Whether one chooses to treat those who are actively using or sets some period of sobriety as a prerequisite, drinking behavior must be monitored carefully and specific goals for drinking behavior must be set. Experience suggests that, for active drinkers who meet criteria for alcohol dependence, an intensive inpatient or partial day treatment program targeting alcohol use is often a good prerequisite or, at least corequisite, for treatment.

Pending disability claims or other litigation (e.g., Social Security or VA disability, worker's compensation, personal injury litigation) often play a role in clients seeking treatment for PTSD. Clinicians often become frustrated with these clients, whom they perceive as seeking treatment for secondary gain and lacking real incentive for change. Nevertheless, these clients can benefit from therapy when clear limits are set and careful treatment planning and goal setting is offered (Meisler, 1995). Other client characteristics that may influence selection and course of treatment include background knowledge and/or treatment of PTSD, comorbid Axis I disorders (e.g., panic, social phobia, major depressive disorder), social supports, and cognitive function. These factors are likely to affect goal setting and pace of progress in treatment.

Inpatient and Outpatient Issues

The treatment program outlined here is designed for use primarily in outpatient settings. As inpatient treatment has increasingly become short-term and crisis-oriented, the focus of treatment must move to outpatient. However, for those who work in acute inpatient settings, the treatment program outlined here can be tailored easily to fit these needs. Two approaches work particularly well. First, after careful assessment of PTSD, substance use, and comorbid disorders, inpatient treatment can focus on many of the earlier stages of treatment, particularly psychoeducation and skill building components. A second and very effective way of applying this program to the inpatient setting is to have multiple groups running at different times or by different therapists, or both. For example, clients may begin in the psychoeducational components of therapy while beginning to learn self-management skills. Such a program would fit very well into many existing substance abuse treatment programs which already incorporate many of the skills components but lack specific PTSD-focused education and treatment. In this way, clients can receive the maximum amount of treatment in what is usually a very time-limited setting. This also allows clinicians with varying expertise and interest to apply their skills to different components of treatment. If treatment is implemented in inpatient settings, it is vital that a coordinated aftercare plan be in place to continue the work begun during hospitalization. In some settings these services may even be provided by the same clinicians. In most settings, however, some collaborative work will be needed to implement this effectively.

Treatment Phases

The following sections outline and describe the essential components of group therapy with PTSD alcohol abusers. These components can be thought of as stages or phases of treatment, with some materials preceding others in a treatment sequence. In general, psychoeducation provides the cornerstone for the treatment, followed by self-management skills training, social skills training and, in some cases, exposure. Motivational enhancement is also an important component of treatment and is woven throughout the other modules. It is important to recognize that although this outline represents a model for treatment, these stages need not be invariant across settings, client populations, or individuals. Individual assessment will reveal areas of relative strength and weakness of each client vis-à-vis the treatment program. Moreover, although a staged approach to treatment is informed by the transtheoretical model (Prochaska & DiClemente, 1982), the model does not dictate how or in what sequence treatment is provided.

There are several overarching features of treatment which span treatment modules.

• Membership of six to eight clients is ideal, although the group may run with as few as four or as many as ten. Although closed groups facilitate peer support and trust, in many settings therapists may choose to open the group when starting a new module which can be offered on a rotating basis.

• Toxicology screens and breathalyzers should be conducted routinely. Refusal to give a specimen or be breathalyzed must always be interpreted as a positive (i.e., *dirty*) result. Clients are instructed not to come to group intoxicated, and are asked to leave if they do so—as long as it is deemed clinically safe (i.e., the client is not suicidal, or, if grossly impaired, has safe means of transportation).

• Each module and each session begin with a brief check-in to inquire about pressing issues, including suicidality, homicidality, and relapse. Check-in also provides clients the opportunity to discuss homework assignments, address difficulties encountered, and receive feedback.

• Clients are instructed to begin daily home monitoring of drinking behavior in the first week of treatment and continue throughout treatment. Monitoring itself can reduce drinking behavior, provide important clinical data about triggers and consequences, and provide a measure of outcome.

- Each module begins with a rationale based both on PTSD and alcohol abuse management. Treatment modules may take one session or span multiple sessions, depending on a number of factors, including client selection, overall length of treatment, and therapist preference.

- Each session includes didactic material, discussion, and skill rehearsal.

TREATMENT MODULES

Psychoeducation about PTSD and Alcohol

Education about alcohol, its acute pharmacologic effects and the sequelae associated with long-term use, is important information that must be conveyed early in treatment. Such information is readily available in video, booklet, and through other sources. If in doubt, check with your local substance abuse treatment facility or the National Institute on Alcohol Abuse and Alcoholism.

Education about alcohol's effects on symptoms and functions related to PTSD is particularly important for engagement at this stage of therapy. Many patients seeking treatment for PTSD may minimize the hazards associated with drinking if they are presented without relevant context. Thus, carefully crafted psychoeducation about the interaction between alcohol's effects and PTSD symptoms can be crucial in engaging patients in active treatment, building alliance, and enhancing motivation. Such education, although initiated early in treatment, continues throughout treatment, serving as a factor in ongoing motivational enhancement. Facts about alcohol that are particularly relevant for individuals with PTSD include the following:

- Alcohol is a depressant. Although it may improve mood in the short run, it increases depression associated with PTSD.

- Alcohol interferes with normal sleep cycles. Although it may assist sleep onset and reduce nightmares by reducing REM, it further impairs the body's normal sleep patterns which are already impaired by PTSD. Frequent attempts to abstain from alcohol, characteristic of dependence, can precipitate REM rebound and exacerbate nightmares. Alcohol abuse causes this vicious cycle of PTSD exacerbation.

- Alcohol narrows attention. Although it sometimes aids in blocking out trauma-related thoughts, at other times it can exacerbate reexperiencing symptoms. Discussion of clients' experience with exaggerated intrusive symptoms during intoxication can be prompted here.

- Alcohol use leads to dependence on alcohol for coping with stress in day-to-day life. Alcohol use will interfere with learning and using the tools and strategies needed to cope with PTSD.

- Withdrawal from alcohol mimics PTSD symptoms (anxiety, hypervigilance, startle, sleep disturbance), leading to a vicious cycle (cf. Saladin, Brady, Dansky, & Kilpatrick, 1995). Alcohol withdrawal should not be mistaken for exacerbation of PTSD symptoms. The spiral of PTSD symptoms, alcohol use, alcohol withdrawal, and symptom exacerbation is illustrated in Figure 7.1

- Physiological and biochemical changes resulting from alcohol cessation can persist for months, resulting in disturbances in sleep, appetite, energy, mood and other functions long after detoxification is complete.

The concept that alcohol not only is harmful in and of itself but also exacerbates PTSD is motivating for many patients. However, some patients may deny that they have experienced any of these harmful effects, particularly those in early stages of recovery or those whose alcohol use disorder has been less severe or disabling. Most patients in group, however, will be able to relate to one or more of these facts about alcohol and PTSD. Facilitate discussion by prompting patients for examples from their own experience.

Date/Time	Trigger	Mood	PTSD sxs (1–10) Pre	Alcohol Craving (1–10) Pre	Strategy used	PTSD sxs (1–10) Post	Alcohol Craving (1–10) Post

Figure 7.1. Sample Home Monitoring Form

Sleep Hygiene

Instruction in and discussion of sleep hygiene is an important part of therapy for PTSD substance abusers. Virtually all clients will rate sleep disturbance as a primary complaint, and many have developed maladaptive methods for coping with these disturbances (e.g., drinking to pass out, taking sedative/hypnotic/anxiolytic medications which lead to dependence, altering sleep cycles to sleep during the day when they feel safer). Important elements of sleep hygiene include:

- Establishing a bedtime routine.

- Avoiding caffeinated beverages after 4 p.m.

- Use of warm baths, warm milk, herbal teas.

- Use of white noise.

- Use of night lights. Darkness is often a conditioned stimulus associated with trauma, and can exacerbate disorientation related to nightmares.

- Relaxation procedures (see below).

Motivational Enhancement

Motivation enhancement represents a set of techniques that are used throughout treatment, though their use early in treatment is particularly important. Capitalizing on clients' motivation for change and enhancing that motivation are key ingredients in the early stages of treatment. In contrast to more traditional approaches to treating addictions which rely on confrontation to deal with resistance and motivate clients, more recent approaches have viewed resistance or ambivalence regarding change as normal and as an appropriate target for therapeutic intervention. Miller & Rollnick (1991) describe a variety of strategies and approaches for enhancing motivation for change. Although the emphasis has been primarily on individual interviewing, many of the same principles are readily applied in the group format.

Express Empathy   Miller and Rollnick (1991) described empathy as an "essential and defining characteristic" of motivational work. Acceptance and understanding of the client's feelings of distress, reasons for drinking, and ambivalence regarding change are vital in the establishment of rapport and trust which are prerequisites for successful use of therapy. Clinicians who are well-versed in PTSD and knowledgeable about the relationship between PTSD and substance use can use this knowledge to facilitate change by allowing the client to feel understood. Clients have often been misunderstood by their family, friends, and even themselves. Many are confused or terrified by their symptoms and fear losing control. Empathy helps to validate the client's experience and thereby facilitates change. Carefully drawn comparisons and analogies among group members' experiences can serve to increase this feeling of understanding, though care must be taken not to exaggerate similarities the client may not see and thereby have the opposite effect.

Develop Discrepancy   Once empathy is established, discrepancy is used in place of direct confrontation. In developing discrepancy, contrasts are drawn between where persons are and where they have stated they want to be. Most clients seeking treatment already perceive the discrepancy; it is often what has led them to therapy in the first place. The clinician amplifies this discrepancy and in doing so increases incentive for change.

Avoid Argumentation   Traditional substance abuse approaches emphasize clients' acceptance of labels such as *alcoholic.* Motivational enhancement approaches avoid confrontation over labels. This principle is particularly important for individuals with PTSD, who often feel the need to control some aspect of their life. Ironically, while many clients may resist the label of alcoholism, a diagnosis of PTSD is often readily accepted, as it provides a schema for understanding their difficulties and can be reassuring. In either case, argumentation over diagnoses, need for treatment, or other issues is counterproductive. The emphasis must be on creating a collaborative spirit in treatment.

Roll with Resistance   Miller and Rollnick (1991) discuss the motivational "judo" that is often helpful in enhancing incentive for change. Resistance and ambivalence regarding change are common and natural, and do not necessarily reflect deep-rooted conflicts. Resistance to change is reflected in many forms in group work with PTSD alcohol abusers, including argumentation, externalization and blame, pessimism, and frank denial. By using empathy and discrepancy along with other techniques (e.g., amplified reflection, reframing), such change-resisting behaviors and the motives that drive them can be minimized and the energy behind them can be converted to more positive, change-enhancing behaviors.

Support Self-Efficacy   Bolstering self-efficacy is essential if change is to occur. Clients may perceive there is a problem and be made aware of strategies for change, but belief in their own ability to carry out change is a key to success. Very often clients "fail" in therapy because they perceive the demands of treatment to be too great. They lack the confidence in their capacity to do the homework, practice the skills, and face their traumatic history, especially without the cushion of alcohol.

Little has been written about the use of motivational techniques such as these in a group therapy format. Most often, these strategies have been employed in the early stages of individual assessment and treatment planning. However, motivational techniques are vital in dealing with ambivalence that surfaces and resurfaces throughout the course of therapy.

Self-Management Skills

Self-management skills comprise the group of skills and tools individuals use to manage their emotional and behavioral responses to internal and external stimuli.

Problem-Solving Individuals with comorbid PTSD and alcohol use disorders frequently lack the skills needed to solve everyday problems of living. Often these deficits develop over time as a function of reliance on avoidant coping strategies associated with both PTSD and substance use. Fear, anxiety, isolation, and depression associated with PTSD further erode problem-solving skills. Problem-solving training in a group therapy format has been shown to be effective in treating other psychiatric patients with substance use disorders (e.g., Carey, Carey, & Meisler, 1990), and it has been emphasized as an important component in therapy with substance abusing PTSD patients in a VA hospital (Abueg & Fairbank, 1992). Problem-solving therapy involves teaching clients a systematic method for identifying and addressing problems in their lives by dividing the process into five distinct components, based on D'Zurilla (1986). These are: problem recognition (acknowledging there is a problem); problem identification (specifying the problem); generating solutions (brainstorming); evaluating alternative solutions (weighing the pros and cons of each); and implementing a plan of action. Each component is introduced and discussed. At each stage of the process, sample problems and problems from clients' own experiences are used for practice of the problem-solving steps. Therapist skill is important here in facilitating problem-solving by guiding appropriate framing and definition of problems. Often, clients will offer problems that appear insurmountable and then use this as a rationale for discounting "problem-solving" as ineffective. For example, the client who states that her problem revolves around her abusive relationship with a partner and her lifelong feelings of low self-worth should be coaxed to reframe the problem into smaller, bite-size chunks which can then be processed. Reframing of problems into manageable pieces and facilitation of brainstorming alternative solutions is critical to problem-solving work with this population. Once action plans are established, supporting self-efficacy to carry out plans and assess outcomes is accomplished through group support and feedback.

Relaxation Skills Relaxation skills are an important part of self-management in any stress or anxiety disorder. Clients are first provided with information about the fight or flight reaction and the physical, cognitive, and emotional effects of chronic hyperarousal. Information about catecholamine alterations in PTSD are also discussed, and clients are asked to discuss ways in which they can tell when they are becoming hyperaroused (e.g., physical sensations). The procedure itself is modeled after the progressive relaxation techniques described by Bernstein & Borkovec (1973). Clients are instructed in the three essential components of relaxation training in sequence. First, diaphragmatic breathing skills are demonstrated and practiced. Second, clients are instructed in progressive muscle relaxation using a seven-muscle-group protocol: forehead; mouth and chin; neck, back, shoulders; legs (nondominant, dominant); arms (nondominant, dominant). Finally, a significant amount of time is spent discussing positive relaxing imagery, including creating safety imagery and dealing with negative or traumatic imagery if it occurs during relaxation. Because the perception of loss of control associated with relaxation can be particularly distressing for clients with PTSD, careful attention is paid to increased feelings of vulnerability among group members, and strategies for remaining in control while permitting relaxation are emphasized. Clients are given tapes and encouraged to practice relaxation skills daily at home.

Anger Management   Irritability, anger, and outright rage are frequent and extremely disabling arousal symptoms of PTSD. Anger also plays a role in many alcohol relapse situations (Marlatt & Gordon, 1985). For many clients with PTSD, anger is experienced as an automatic reaction to a variety of events. This can be explained in part by conditioned arousal reactions to threatening stimuli. This poses a challenge to the cognitive model of anger proposed in many therapies, in which the connection between events and behavior is mediated by thoughts and beliefs. Therefore, treatment must emphasize the importance of stress reducing relaxation procedures. A threshold model is used to help explain the importance of keeping arousal below the boiling point. By slowing down such reactivity, intervention becomes possible. Clients are first asked to discuss examples of angry behavior and of ways in which anger and aggression has caused problems in their lives. The positive, life-protecting effects of anger are also discussed, with reemphasis of the fight or flight response discussed previously. Clients are introduced to the concept of triggers, and discuss anger triggers in their lives. They are instructed to keep a log of anger situations, the triggers, and both internal (e.g., tension, confusion) and external (e.g., arguments, isolation) consequences. Short-term cooling off strategies are discussed and practiced. Clients are given sample conflict situations as well as examples from their own experience, and group members role play with an emphasis on shaping and guiding anger management strategies.

Self-Reinforcement   As avoidance and alcohol use have replaced many other activities, dually-diagnosed clients often have lost ability to reward themselves for progress they have made, especially without alcohol. Feelings of guilt and anhedonia often interfere. However, as patients gain sobriety and increase coping skills, their ability to reward themselves becomes crucial to increased independence and decreased reliance on alcohol. Exploration of activities and things clients find rewarding is accomplished through discussion. Lists of possible activities can be provided to clients, and assistance in engaging in these activities is offered. Money saved from abstinence from alcohol can be put toward desired things or activities. Occasionally, client consultation with recreation specialists to identify and explore these options is useful.

Cognitive Refocusing   Traumatized clients often find it nearly impossible to distract themselves and refocus when they are having intrusive thoughts and when urges to use alcohol are strong. Symptoms of PTSD can serve as cognitive blinders, narrowing attention onto negative aspects of experience and preventing an adaptive shift in attention. Paradoxically, alcohol use in these conditions may actually accentuate this negative focus (Sayette, Wilson, & Carpenter, 1989). Strategies designed to assist clients in refocusing include traditional thought-stopping techniques, as well as techniques derived from Eastern philosophies, including mindfulness meditation. Linehan (1993) provides a variety of useful "grounding strategies" developed for work with borderline clients, and many transfer well to work with PTSD substance abusers.

Social Skills Training

Social skills comprise the group of skills and behaviors that facilitate interaction with the world in a positive and productive way. Many of these skills are derived from the skills training work with alcohol abusers (e.g., Monti, Abrams, Kadden, & Cooney, 1989). For the dually-diagnosed client, the critical skills that are often lacking revolve around assertiveness and availing themselves of social support. In these modules, the concept is introduced by prompting discussion of situations in which group members may have had difficulty in this type of situation. The rationale for the skill is discussed, instruction is provided, and role play and rehearsal is used to practice and refine the skills.

Assertiveness   Assertiveness is a fundamental skill needed to successfully maintain sobriety. Dually-diagnosed clients often vacillate between avoidance and passivity on the one hand and anger and rage on the other. The topic is introduced by having the group discuss the difference between assertiveness and aggression. Other communication styles, such as passive and passive-aggressive styles, are introduced and discussed. The advantages of assertiveness in gaining control of one's life are discussed. Specific components of assertiveness, such as specificity, directness, and body language are discussed, and the skills are practiced and role played in group. Importantly, individual client barriers to implementing these skills are assessed and discussed in order to facilitate generalization beyond the group.

Drink Refusal Skills   Invitations to drink are inevitable. The ability to refuse such offers is important, particularly in the early stages of sobriety when individuals are highly vulnerable to slips and relapse. As Monti and colleagues (1989) point out, refusal of such offers requires more than simply the desire not to drink; it requires the specific assertiveness skills to carry out that refusal. Clients discuss situations they have encountered or might anticipate in the near future. Drawing on skills learned in the assertiveness module, strategies of saying "no," offering alternatives, and avoiding excuse making are discussed, rehearsed, and role-played.

Receiving Criticism   Clients with PTSD and alcohol problems often respond to criticism with hurt, shame, defensiveness, and anger. Constructive criticism may be perceived as destructive, particularly during active drinking phases. Distinguishing between these types of criticism is reviewed, and clients discuss examples from their experience.

Seeking and Accepting Social Support   Social support is a critical element in achieving sobriety and facing PTSD-related difficulties. For many clients, however, social supports have dwindled as a result of social avoidance, isolation, and drinking. For some, receiving social support may seem threatening, eliciting feelings of vulnerability, guilt, or resentment. Therefore, the module should start with a discussion of existing social supports and perceived barriers to support, including personal, interpersonal, and environmental factors. Different types of support are discussed, such as practical, financial, moral, and so on. As the importance of social support is recognized and discussed, clients begin to identify ways to form and maintain supports. These include broadening networks (e.g., AA), using assertiveness skills to request support when needed, and learning basic communication and support skills of one's own that are instrumental in establishing supportive relationships.

Relapse Prevention

A great deal has been written on the topic of relapse prevention (e.g., Marlatt & Gordon, 1985). It is an integral part of all cognitive-behavioral treatment programs for substance abuse, and the application of the techniques to individuals with PTSD and comorbid substance use disorders has been well described (e.g., Abueg & Fairbank, 1992). Many of the coping skills needed for effective relapse prevention have already been covered in earlier phases of treatment, as have triggers related to moods and PTSD symptoms that can lead to alcohol use. Thus, during this phase, the focus is on integrating this material and applying it through role play, homework assignments, and group discussion to foster a greater understanding and greater self-efficacy in implementing the knowledge and skills learned. Continued home-monitoring, such as daily use of the chart in Figure 7.2, can assist clients in identifying the way PTSD symptoms might contribute to relapse and how to best use strategies for managing these triggers.

Direct Therapeutic Exposure

It has long been recognized that exposure-based therapies are the treatment of choice for most anxiety disorders, particularly simple phobias and obsessive-compulsive disorder. Studies of exposure treatment for PTSD have also been encouraging (e.g., Foa, Rothbaum, Riggs, & Murdock, 1991; Keane, Fairbank, Caddell, & Zimering, 1989). Moreover, alcohol researchers have found exposure therapy to be useful in treating addictions by combining extinction-based procedures with coping skills training (Monti et al., 1993). However, only now is systematic investigation under way to examine the utility of exposure work in the context of group therapy for PTSD (Friedman & Schnurr, 1997), and to date no reports of group exposure work with substance abusers is available. In fact, substance use is often cited as an exclusion for exposure work (e.g., Litz, Blake, Gerardi, & Keane, 1990). Nevertheless, given the association of trauma and alcohol cues in the dually-diagnosed, an exposure therapy that incorporates both types of cues merits investigation. Clinically, these concepts can be applied in the later phases of treatment by having group members engage in imaginal exposure of high risk scenes including both trauma and alcohol cues and using various skills learned in treatment to reduce subjective distress and craving. Repeated guided covert exposure to these cues can result in reduced arousal, reduced craving, and increased self-efficacy.

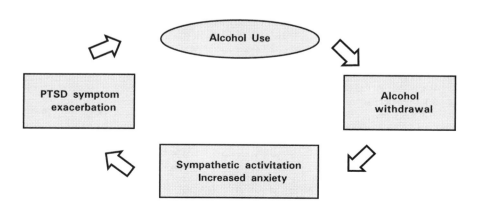

Figure 7.2. Cycle of PTSD and Alcohol Withdrawal

Additional Treatment Components

For many clients, group therapy will be more effective as part of a comprehensive treatment package. For example, AA meetings can provide additional support and encouragement in achieving and maintaining sobriety, although a number of clients with PTSD may find certain aspects of AA philosophy troubling (Satel, Becker, & Dan, 1993). Individual, couples, or family therapy, or both, may also be necessary in addition to group treatment. Involvement in these therapies should not be exclusions for group participation provided that communication between group therapists and other treaters is open and opportunities for splitting and fractionation of care are minimized. Pharmacologic management is likely to be useful, particularly for depressed clients who find participation in group work and homework assignments overwhelming. The use of antabuse and naloxone/naltrexone can also provide important adjuncts to group treatment.

CONCLUSION

Group therapy for individuals with PTSD and comorbid alcohol use disorders is an exciting and important treatment modality. Development and empirical validation of these approaches are in their infancy, and much additional work is needed. Although many of the techniques described here have been used with other clinical populations (e.g., substance abusers), their application and refinement with the dually-diagnosed represents an important advance. Use of these modalities in conjunction with the collection of process and outcome data will enhance our ability to deliver effective group therapy for individuals with PTSD and alcohol use disorders.

REFERENCES

Abueg, F. R., & Fairbank, J. A. (1992). Behavioral treatment of post-traumatic stress disorder and co-occurring substance abuse. In P. A. Saigh (Ed.), *Post-traumatic stress disorder: A behavioral approach to assessment and treatment.* Boston: Allyn & Bacon.

Bernstein, D. A., & Borkovec, T. D. (1973). *Progressive relaxation training.* Champaign, IL: Research Press.

Carey, M. P., Carey, K. B., & Meisler, A. W. (1990). Training mentally ill chemical abusers in social problem-solving. *Behavior Therapy, 21,* 511–518.

Charney, D. S., Deutch, A. Y., Krystal, J. H., Southwick, S. M., & Davis, M. (1993). Psychobiologic mechanisms of post-traumatic stress disorder. *Archives of General Psychiatry, 50,* 294–305.

Cooney, N. L., Baker, L. H., Pomerleau, O. F., & Josephy, B. (1984). Salivation to drinking cues in alcohol abusers: Toward the validation of a physiological measure of craving. *Addictive Behaviors, 9,* 91–94.

Cottler, L. B., Compton, W. M., Mager, D., Spitznagel, E. L., & Janca, A. (1992). Post-traumatic stress disorder among substance users from the general population. American *Journal of Psychiatry, 149,* 664–670.

Drake, R. E., & Noordsy, D. L. (1996). Case management for people with coexisting severe mental disorder and substance use disorder. In N. Miller (Ed.), *Addiction psychiatry.* New York: W. B. Saunders.

D'Zurilla, T. J. (1986). *Problem-solving therapy: A social competence approach to clinical intervention.* New York: Springer.

Foa, E. B., Rothbam, B. O., Riggs, D. S., & Murdock, T. B. (1991). Treatment of post-traumatic stress disorder in rape victims: A comparison between cognitive–behavioral procedures and counseling. *Journal of Consulting and Clinical Psychology, 59,* 715–723.

Fontana, A., Rosenheck, R., Spencer, H., & Gray, S. (1995). *The long journey home IV: The fourth progress report on the department of veterans affairs specialized PTSD programs.* West Haven, CT: Department of Veterans Affairs, Northeast Program Evaluation Center.

Friedman, M. J., & Schnurr, P. P. (1997). *Department of Veterans Affairs VA cooperative study #420: Group treatment of PTSD.* White River Junction, VT: National Center for PTSD.

Fullilove, M. T., Fullilove, R. E., Smith, M., Winkler, K., Michael, C., Panzer, P. G., & Wallace, R. (1993). Violence, trauma, and post-traumatic stress disorder among women drug users. *Journal of Traumatic Stress, 6,* 533–543.

Green, B. L., Lindy, J. D., Grace, M. C., & Gleser, G. C. (1989). Multiple diagnoses in post-traumatic stress disorder: The role of war stressors. *Journal of Nervous and Mental Disease, 177,* 329–335.

Keane, T. M., Fairbank, J. A., Caddell, J. M., & Zimering, R. T. (1989). Implosive (flooding) therapy reduces symptoms of PTSD in Vietnam combat veterans. *Behavior Therapy, 20,* 245–260.

Keane, T. M., Gerardi, R. J., Lyons, J. A., & Wolfe, J. (1988). The interrelationship of substance abuse and post-traumatic stress disorder: Epidemiological and clinical considerations. In M. Galanter (Ed.), *Recent developments in alcoholism* (vol. 6). New York: Plenum.

Keane, T. M., & Kaloupek, D. G. (1982). Imaginal flooding in the treatment of post-traumatic stress disorder. *Journal of Consulting and Clinical Psychology, 50,* 138–140.

Khantzian, E. J. (1985). The self-medication hypothesis of addictive disorders: Focus on heroin and cocaine dependence. *American Journal of Psychiatry, 143,* 1259–1264.

Lacousiere, R. B., Godfrey, K. B., & Ruby, L. M. (1980). Traumatic neurosis in the etiology of alcoholism: Vietnam combat and other trauma. *American Journal of Psychiatry, 137,* 966–968.

Levenson, R. W., Sher, K., Grossman., L., Newman, J., & Newlin, D. (1980). Alcohol and stress response dampening: Pharmacological effects, expectancy, and tension reduction. *Journal of Abnormal Psychology, 89,* 528–538.

Linehan, M. M. (1993). *Skills training manual for treating borderline personality disorder.* New York: Guilford.

Litz, B. T., Blake, D. D., Gerardi, R. G., & Keane, T. M. (1990). Decision making guidelines for the use of direct therapeutic exposure in the treatment of post-traumatic stress disorder. *Behavior Therapist, 13,* 91–93.

Marlatt, G. A., & Gordon, J. R. (1985). *Relapse prevention: Maintenance strategies in the treatment of addictive behaviors.* New York: Guilford.

McFall, M. E., McKay, P. W., & Donovan, D. M. (1992). Combat-related post-traumatic stress disorder and severity of substance abuse in Vietnam veterans. *Journal of Studies on Alcohol, 53,* 357–363.

Meisler, A. W. (1995, September). Disability benefits and the clinician: Problems and challenges. In S. W. Southwick (Chair), Do *disability benefits make patients sicker?* New Haven, CT: Yale University School of Medicine.

Meisler, A. W. (1996a). Trauma, PTSD, and substance abuse. *PTSD Research Quarterly, 7*(4), 1–6.

Meisler, A. W. (1996b, November). PTSD and substance abuse in Vietnam combat veterans: Behavioral theroy, research, and practice. Paper in L. M. Najavits (Chair), *Post-traumatic stress disorder and substance abuse: New clinical frontiers.* Symposium presented at the annual meeting of the International Society for Traumatic Stress Studies, San Francisco, CA.

Miller, W. R., & Rollnick, S. (1991). *Motivational interviewing: Preparing people to change addictive behaviors.* New York: Guilford.

Monti, P. M., Abrams, D. B., Kadden, R. M., & Cooney, N. L. (1989). *Treating alcohol dependence.* New York: Guilford.

Monti, P. M., Binkoff, J. A., Abrams, D. B., Zwick, W. R., Nirenberg, T. D., & Liepman, M. R. (1987). Reactivity of alcoholics and nonalcoholics to drinking cues. *Journal of Abnormal Psychology, 96,* 122–126.

Monti, P. M., Rohsenow, D. J., Rubonis, A. V., Niaura, R. S., Sirota, A. D., Colby, S. M., Goddard, P., & Abrams, D. B. (1993). Cue exposure with coping skills treatment for male alcoholics: A preliminary investigation. *Journal of Consulting and Clinical Psychology, 61,* 1011–1019.

Najavits, L. M., Weiss, R. D., & Liese, B. S. (1996). Group cognitive-behavioral therapy for women with PTSD and substance use disorder. *Journal of Substance Abuse Treatment, 13,* 13–22.

Najavits, L. M., Weiss, R. D., & Shaw, S. R. (1996, November). Outcome of a new manualized cognitive-behavioral therapy for women with PTSD and substance abuse. In L. M. Najavits (Chair), *Post-traumatic stress disorder and substance abuse: New clinical frontiers.* Symposium presented at the annual meeting of the International Society for Traumatic Stress Studies, San Francisco.

Orr, S. (1994). An overview of psychophysiological studies of PTSD. *PTSD Research Quarterly, 5*(1), 1–7.

Padin-Rivera, E., Donovan, B. S., & McCormick, R. A. (1996). *Transcend: A treatment program for veterans with post-traumatic stress disorder and substance abuse disorders.* Unpublished document, VA Medical Center, Cleveland, OH.

Prochaska, J. O., & DiClemente, C. C. (1982). Transtheoretical therapy: Toward a more integrative model of change. *Psychotherapy: Theory, Research, and Practice, 19,* 276–288.

Reifman, A., & Windle, M. (1996). Vietnam combat exposure and recent drug use: A national study. *Journal of Traumatic Stress, 9,* 557–568.

Saladin, M. E., Brady, K. T., Dansky, B. S., & Kilpatrick, D. G. (1995). Understanding comorbidity between PTSD and substance use disorders: Two preliminary investigations. *Addictive Behaviors, 20,* 643–655.

Salkovskis, P. M., & Reynolds, M. (1994). Thought suppression and smoking cessation. *Behaviour Research and Therapy, 32,* 193–201.

Sayette, M. A., Wilson, G. T., & Carpenter, J. A. (1989). Cognitive moderators of alcohol's effects on anxiety. *Behaviour Research and Therapy, 27,* 685–690.

Satel, S. L., Becker, B. R., & Dan, E. (1993). Reducing obstacles to affiliation with Alcoholics Anonymous among veterans with PTSD and alcoholism. *Hospital and Community Psychiatry, 44,* 1061–1065.

Stewart, S. H. (1996). Alcohol abuse in individuals exposed to trauma: A critical review. *Psychological Bulletin, 120,* 83–112.

Tunis, S. L., Deluchi, K. L., & Hall, S. M. (1994). Assessing thoughts about cocaine and their relationship to short-term treatment outcome. *Experimental and Clinical Psychopharmacology, 2,* 184–193.

Chapter 8

Supportive Group Therapy for Bereavement After Homicide

E.K. Rynearson and Cindi S. Sinnema

INTRODUCTION

A recent study of a representative sample of 2,181 persons aged 18 to 45 years in the Detroit area assessed the lifetime hsitory of traumatic events and PTSD, according to DSM-IV (Breslau, Kessler, Chilcoat, Schultz, Craig, & Andreski, 1998). These researchers found that sudden unexpected death of a loved one is a far more important cause of PTSD in the community than rape and other assaultive violence, accounting for nearly one third of PTSD cases. In another recent study, PTSD symptoms were found among residents of a community exposed to serial murder, suggesting even "indirect" violence can result in severe psychological distress (Herkov & Biernat, 1997).

Supportive group therapy arose for bereaved family members whose loved ones were murdered amidst the advent of numerous support groups emerging in the 1970s. Homicide support groups were generally informal gatherings intended to provide mutual support during the criminal investigation and trial, and to share experiences about how their lives had been affected.

Over time, homicide support groups have become more structured. Two particularly excellent books offer detailed descriptions of support group therapy (Redmond, 1989; Spungen, 1998). Moreover, studies of systematic interventions are beginning to appear in the literature. Murphy, Baugher, Lohan, Scheideman, Heerwagen, Johnson, Tillery, & Grover (1996) reviewed 156 bereaved parents' evaluations of a two-dimensional support program for parents whose children died by accident, homicide, or suicide. Both problem-focused support and emotion-focused support were reported to be effective.

A more recent study (Murphy, Johnson, Das Gupta, Cain, Dimond, Lohan, & Baugher, in press), the first controlled study of intervention effects after homicide, similarly looked at 261 parents of children who died by accident, homicide, or suicide. Participants were randomly assigned to control or intervention groups (a 10-session weekly 2-hour education support group). Data were collected at pre- and postintervention/control assignment and 6 months later. Highly distressed mothers showed a significant response—fathers and less distressed mothers showed no significant change with intervention. Parents of homicidal death were more highly distressed than parents of accidental or suicidal death. These findings suggest that mothers of homicide victims are the most vulnerable to stress and the most responsive to support group intervention.

Over 20 years ago, I (EKR) attended my first support group for family members after a homicidal death. Like most support groups, it arose spontaneously from the members' determination to help one another. It was held in the living room of one of the group's leaders. About 20 of us sat in a circle drinking coffee, while a large plate of homemade cookies was passed among us. Each member's introduction was followed by a brief telling of the homicidal tragedy that brought them to this place. A young, tremulous woman began her introduction by saying that this was her first meeting, and it was to be her last. She was very sorry, but she could not stand hearing these "awful stories." She burst into tears as she fled toward the safety of her car. The leader followed her out. When he returned, he reassured us that he would call her later that night. The next member then launched into a bitter monologue about the incompetence of the police, courts, and the prison system, demanding that this group actively lobby the legislature to pressure for change. An older couple then thanked the group for listening to them the month before at the last meeting. They looked forward to returning because there seemed to be a unique empathy from other family members who could resonate and reflect with them about their daughter's homicidal death.

I remember walking towards my car after we said our goodbyes, feeling perplexed by what seemed so discordant about the meeting; the painful narratives of homicide by everyone, the nurturance and empathy of some members, the strident demands for action by others, and the frightened exit of the young woman. She had parked in front of me, and I could see her skid marks in my headlights. I worried that the support group had further traumatized her.

Thereafter, I volunteered to serve as a consultant for the organization. I was enlivened by their altruism and emboldened by their hope that they could help. The support group was their only collective offering. Most of their outreach was through individual phone calls, home visits, or individual advocacy during interviews with the media, the police, and court proceedings, but the monthly support group was the centerpiece of their recovery program. There was never an agenda, and I soon learned that there was no systematic model followed by the leader.

Though they met only once a month, there was no limit to the number of sessions one attended. Like most support groups, there were eight or ten long-term members who had no intention of leaving. There seemed to be a mixture of factors responsible for their fixity. Long-term recovery required: long-term support for some; chronic anger, distrust, and demands for retribution for a few; and a characterologic assumption of the role of victim for several. Obviously, these long-term members had differing assumptions about what would be helpful. The themes of empathy, strident activism, and masochism seemed intrusive instead of integrative to me. There was a procession of newer members who would attend for six or eight sessions, and then leave the group with a stirring testimonial.

I attended this group for two years after which I wrote one of the early descriptive studies of homicidal bereavement (Rynearson, 1984). At that point, I was attempting to differentiate this traumatic bereavement process from the more familiar bereavement after a natural death. I tentatively suggested that trauma distress and separation distress were combined reactions after an unnatural death. In later papers (Rynearson, 1986, 1987), I suggested a preliminary conceptual model of bereavement after unnatural dying, and in more recent papers (Rynearson, 1994; Rynearson & McCreery, 1993), I have speculated about the mechanisms of recovery and treatment. Though I have consistently led support groups composed of family members after unnatural death, it has been in the last five years only that I have become more specific in establishing a protocol.

Before detailing these guidelines for supportive group psychotherapy, I will outline a conceptual model underlying these recommendations.

CONCEPTUAL MODEL OF TRAUMATIC BEREAVEMENT

The bereavement following an unnatural death summons two concurrent distress responses: separation distress as a response to the lost relationship, and trauma distress to the manner of dying. While these distress responses are admixed, they maintain as distinct syndromes arising from either death itself (separation distress) or unnatural dying (traumatic distress). Table 8.1 outlines their descriptive categorization.

TABLE 8.1.

	Trauma Distress	Separation Distress
Thoughts	Reenactment	Reunion
Feelings	Fear	Longing
Behavior	Avoidance	Searching

The reader will recognize that this categorization cannot be clinically applied with rigorous accuracy or discrimination in every subject. The diverse responses of family members during bereavement will challenge any categorization. This model, however, suggests that bereavement is a multidimensional process rather than a model of epigenetic stages or unconscious forces. Further, the model of concurrent trauma and separation distress may be applied with both natural and unnatural dying since some degree of trauma distress is associated with a direct experience of death itself. Figure 8.1 illustrates a hypothetical plotting of trauma and separation distress with natural dying and Figure 8.2 does the same for unnatural dying.

This model presumes that unrecovered family members after an unnatural death will present with sustained trauma distress that overshadows separation distress. The model presumes that trauma distress takes neuropsychologic precedence over separation distress in its expression and in treatment as well.

SUPPORT PROJECT FOR UNNATURAL DYING

In 1990, we established a community outreach program for each family in the greater Seattle area following a homicide. With the collaborative support of the medical examiner's office, the police, prosecuting attorney's office, victims' assistance agencies, and mental health services, we offered supportive intervention.

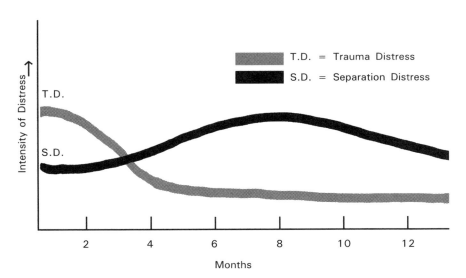

Figure 8.1. Natural Death

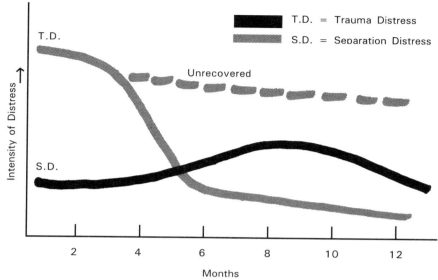

Figure 8.2.   Natural Death

During the past seven years, we have worked with nearly 250 family members. Our theoretical and practical approach to their recovery in large part has evolved from clinical attunement. Intervention begins with a home visit. On the basis of that visit, which includes a 60-minute semistructured interview and measures of trauma, depression, and substance abuse, we offer several alternatives for assistance.

We have developed an algorithm that illustrates the direction and staging of interventions (see Figure 8.3).

Screening Process

Family members are identified through the medical examiner's office, which allows us access to its listing of homicidal deaths. Within the first two months of the homicide, we contact the family with a letter offering our support and offering a home visit for further assistance. On average, four months have passed since the homicide before we make the home visit. A semistructured interview follows during which we check for risk factors for nonrecovery: Previous psychiatric disorder and treatment; presence of comorbid psychiatric disorders at the time of interview; and the presence of intense, traumatic distress with signs of intense avoidance and intrusive reenactment imagery (Rynearson, 1995). The presence of one or more of these risk factors recommends an alternative intervention before entering a support group.

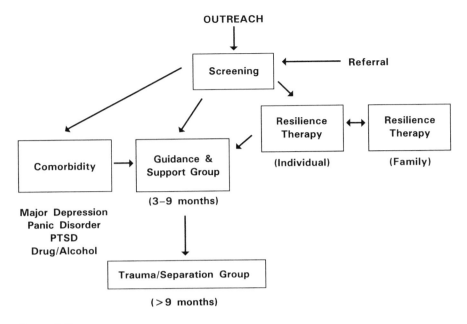

Figure 8.3

Resilience Therapy for Trauma Distress

While intrusive imagery and avoidant behavior are common during the first month of bereavement, they spontaneously moderate in the vast majority of family members. When signs and symptoms of trauma distress continue on a daily basis for four to six months, it becomes disruptive. Several (average four to six) weekly individual sessions to reinforce self-calming with relaxation techniques and encourage thought diversion with guided imagery can diminish arousal and terror. Rather than focusing on the dying imagery an active inquiry of the previous life pattern of the deceased is begun. Participants are encouraged to bring family picture albums so vivified imagery of the deceased can counterbalance the traumatic death imagery. In our experience, this active psychotherapeutic technique of a nurturant reconstruction of the internalized image of the deceased seems to diminish avoidance and enhance engagement and alliance in recovery.

Involving other family members in a modified family therapy to reinforce resilient capacities and support may also be indicated. Educating all family members that the nonverbal capacities of resilience are crucial in early recovery will help them as well. Without these capacities for resilience (self-calming, self-differentiation, and self-transcendence) it will be difficult for the family to maintain its cohesion and commitment to one another (Rynearson, 1996).

Psychiatric Consultation

At any point, psychiatric consultation will be considered if the family member meets criteria for comorbid psychiatric disorder. In our five-year study, 60% of family members who sought therapy were referred for psychiatric consultation. Major depression, anxiety disorders, post-traumatic stress syndrome (PTSD) and substance abuse most often presented in combination rather than pure form. Pharmacotherapy and substance abuse therapy were combined with the psychotherapeutic interventions.

Guidance and Support Group

Our observations of family members during the first year of adjustment after a homicide revealed their initial preoccupation with the media and the criminal judicial system. During the first six to twelve months, they are swept along by the cultural-social demand that the crime be publicly exposed and that the murderer be found and punished, which promises revenge for the victim and retribution for the family. Unfortunately, this cultural-social proscription promises more than it delivers. The family member has little choice but to cooperate. The media, the investigators, and eventually the court, if the murderer is found, need something from the family member (e.g., testimonial details of the victim's past and present history to explain the homicide). They each have a job to do. Their commitment to the family member is necessarily short-term and not primarily concerned with their well-being.

Because of this wave of social scrutiny and inquest, we have tried to provide support that includes abundant definition and clarification of these social demands and the rights of family members. We have designed a time-limited group program with a proscribed agenda of topics highly relevant to the first six to twelve months of adjustment (see Table 8.2). We believe it is reassuring to family members to sense that we can offer a pragmatic service that will provide a more coherent understanding of this enforced social ordeal while reinforcing their social rights and autonomy. Some of the topics include clinical issues of comorbidity, family support, and crime victims' funding. These are clinical topics that have particular relevance in the initial phase of recovery. They also alert group members to risk factors and early signs of nonrecovery to make them more accepting of alternate intervention. Sometimes they are able to identify these harbingers of nonrecovery in other family members who might want to be included in therapy. Every session includes written descriptive handouts which reinforce clarification and discussion. Family members are included during one of the last sessions to educate and engage them as well.

Group members are invited to repeat another 10 sessions if that would be of support. It is not unusual to start a group with five or six new members and three or

TABLE 8.2   Guidance and Support Group

Session 1	**Introduction of Members** **Focus:** Sharing stories.
Session 2	**Focus:** What is grief? Physical and emotional manifestations of grief.
Session 3	**Focus:** Differing grief styles. Exploring uniqueness based on age, history, relationships, and family experience.
Session 4	**Focus:** Self-care including: commemoration of special days and choosing a therapist.
Session 5	**Focus:** Criminal justice process: how a typical homicide investigation works, common elements and timeline of a trial and definitions of common legal terms and procedures.
Session 6	**Focus:** Impact of the criminal justice system on grief. Expectations and reality are often different. How can we reconcile these differences?
Session 7	**Focus:** Gender and grief. The impact of grief on men and women. How do these differences impact relationships?
Session 8	**Focus:** Family night. How families and individuals grieve differently. Sharing family pictures.
Session 9	**Focus:** Exploring faith and spirituality questions. Is the world a safe place? Why do bad things happen? Why us? What do I believe?
Session 10	**Focus:** Last group session. Reflections

four members who want to remain for further support. We have never had anyone repeat more than twice and the drop out rate has been remarkably low.

Trauma and Separation Distress Group

We offer a support group with a different agenda and objectives after nine to twelve months of recovery. By this time, the public scrutiny and inquest will have passed. Like the initial support group, this intervention is time-limited (10 sessions) and follows a prescribed course (see Table 8.3). Most of the members present with persistent and intense trauma distress with heightened avoidance and intrusion. Our initial objective in the early sessions is a clarification of trauma and separation distress while introducing anxiety management and guided imagery to reinforce resilient capacities. Resources of support and concepts of death are explored to compensate for the sense of helplessness and empty nihilism that often accompanies nonrecovery. The group then focuses on the model of dialectic instead of homeostatic recovery, the concept that the homicide has to some extent created a permanent change. Comorbid psychiatric disorders need to be identified and treated since their syndromes may be misinterpreted as unrecovered trauma and separation distress.

The remaining sessions deal more directly with persistent reenactment imagery. Initially, we encourage members to present brief descriptive monologues with pictures, poems, and art to celebrate the life of the deceased. Once this positive imagery is established, we focus on the more horrific imagery of the dying. We ask each of the members to draw out the death scene on a large piece of paper which they then present to the group. With the imagery before us, we can then begin to reprocess their fantasy by including more active fantasies of rescue, reunion, relin-

TABLE 8.3. Trauma/Separation Support Group

Session 1	**Introduction of Members** **Focus:** Clarification of trauma and separation. How can we remain resilient? How have you remained resilient in the past?
Session 2	**Focus:** Resources of support: family, friends, work, spiritual. Who or what was supportive in the past? What is your concept of death?
Session 3	**Focus:** Model of prevailing instead of recovery. How can I accept how I have changed? How can I help others adjust to this change?
Session 4	**Focus:** Obstacles to prevailing: comorbidity, self-blame, and revenge. How do we define and manage comorbidity? How can I deal with self-blame and revenge?
Session 5	**Focus:** Commemorative imagery and narratives: tell a story about the person before the death. Use journal, pictures, poetry, music.
Session 6	**Focus:** Commemorative continued. Preparation for Session 7.
Session 7	**Focus:** Death imagery (to be explained).
Session 8	**Focus:** Death imagery continued.
Session 9	**Focus:** Family session.
Session 10	**Focus:** Session for goodbye or recommitment.

quishment, and sometimes revenge. This rich interchange often includes the last thoughts and feelings of the deceased—and what the surviving family member would have said in response.

Family members rarely ask to repeat this group. The active reprocessing of trauma distress and imagery provides enough relief that they are now able to deal more directly with separation distress on their own. We are available for ongoing support, but this is rarely requested.

CONCLUSION

Supportive group therapy has been a widely applied and clinically useful therapy for family members after an unnatural death. In this chapter, we have presented a model of nonrecovery that suggests that intervention will include supportive group therapy as but one aspect of a more inclusive approach. This model suggests that comorbid psychiatric disorders and intense trauma distress are early risk factors for nonrecovery and need intervention before considering a support group. Since early recovery demands an involvement with the media and the criminal judicial system, we recommend an initial involvement in a time-limited support group with an agenda that focuses on this aftermath with clarification and pragmatic support. Later recovery will deal with the more subjective aftermath of trauma and separation distress for which we would recommend a time-limited support group with a different agenda assisting in the clarification and shared resolution of persistent trauma distress. Individual, family, or psychiatric support may be requested at any point, but these interventions will be time-limited as well.

Maintaining a time-limited and focused format is presumably less threatening to family members after this tragedy than an unstructured program that meets less frequently for many months or years. This format also ensures that family members with long-term support needs that often antedated the unnatural death will not take over a group with their angry demands and outrage over their perceived victimization. These subjects are better served by a long-term commitment from a therapist outside the support program since the recent homicide is only the latest in a procession of traumas that sometimes began in their childhood.

It is important to note that these clinical impressions of our structured program's advantages are just that—clinical impressions. There has been no controlled outcome study to verify these impressions, though we plan on doing such a study in the near future. While our guidelines for supportive group therapy are untested, our experience has demonstrated a high degree of engagement and commitment. Our dropout rate is almost nonexistent (participants tend to drop out because of scheduling problems or actual moves from the area).

We are confident that had this structured program been a basis for that first support group I attended over 20 years ago, new members would have been better prepared. The young woman who fled that first session would have been assessed for the presence of traumatic intrusive imagery and avoidance that prevented her engagement. Once engaged, she would have been offered a definite path of intervention to follow. After an unnatural death, family members need an assurance of coherence and autonomy to counterbalance their terror and helplessness. While our program cannot promise coherence and autonomy, we can at least present a structured pathway through the morass of homicidal bereavement until the family members have found footing on their own path.

REFERENCES

Herkov, M. J., Biernat, M. (1997). Assessment of PTSD symptoms in a community exposed to serial murder. *Journal of Clinical Psychology, 53,* 809–815.

Murphy, S. A., Baugher, R., Lohar, J., Scheideman, J., Heerwagen, J., Johnson, L. C., Tillery, L., & Grover, M. C. (1996). Parents' evaluation of a preventive intervention following the sudden violent deaths of their children. *Death Studies, 20,* 453–468.

Murphy, S. A., Johnson, L. C., Das Gupta, A., Cain, K., Dimond, M., Loha, J., & Baugher, R. (1998). A preventive group intervention for bereaved parents: A randomized controlled trial. *Death Studies, 22,* 1–27.

Redmond, L. M. (1989). *Surviving: When someone you loved was murdered. A professional's guide to group therapy for families and friends of murdered victims.* Clearwater, FL: Psychological Consultation and Education Services.

Rynearson, E. K. (1984). Bereavement after homicide: A descriptive study. *American Journal of Psychiatry, 141,* 1452–1454.

Rynearson, E. K. (1986). Psychological effects of unnatural dying on bereavement. *Psychiatric Annals, 16,* 272–275.

Rynearson, E. K. (1987). Bereavement after unnatural dying. In S. Zisook (Ed.), *Advances in bereavement* (pp. 77–93). Washington, DC: American Psychiatric Press.

Rynearson, E. K. (1994). Psychotherapy of bereavement after homicide. *Journal of Psychotherapy Practice and Research* (Fall), 341–347.

Rynearson, E. K. (1995). Bereavement after homicide. A comparison of treatment seekers and refusers. *British Journal of Psychiatry, 166,* 507–510.

Rynearson, E. K. (1996). Psychotherapy of bereavement after homicide: Be offensive. *In Session: Psychotherapy in Practice, 2,* 47–57.

Rynearson, E. K., & McCreery, J. M. (1993). Bereavement after homicide: A synergism of trauma and loss. *American Journal of Psychiatry, 150,* 258–261.

Spungen, D. (1998). *Homicide: The hidden victims. A guide for professionals.* Thousand Oaks, CA: Sage Publications.

Chapter 9

Cognitive-Behavioral Group Treatment for Disaster-Related PTSD

Bruce H. Young, Josef I. Ruzek, and Julian D. Ford

The extreme and overwhelming forces of disaster often have far-reaching effects on individuals and communities. Though a disaster may last from seconds to several days, its effects may continue from months to years during the process of recovery and restoration. The lack of uniformity of methodology across studies coupled with the inherent difficulties in the study of disaster survivors, make it difficult to draw a definitive conclusion about the wide ranging prevalence rates of PTSD in disaster survivors reported in literature reviews (de Girolamo & McFarlane, 1996; Smith & North, 1993). The experiences of disaster survivors vary greatly, and it is likely that certain kinds of disaster-related experiences (e.g., bereavement, exposure to personal life threat, property loss) put victims at a higher risk for psychological problems (Bland, O'Leary, Farinaro, Jossa, & Revisau, 1996; Bromet, Parkinson, Schulberg, Dunn, & Gondek, 1982; Gleser, Green, & Winget, 1981; Goenjian et al., 1994; Green, Grace, & Gleser, 1985; Green et al., 1992; Keane, Pickett, Jepson, McCorkle, & Lowrey, 1994; Pfifer & Norris, 1989; Shore, Tatum, & Vollmer, 1986).

During the last decade there has been a remarkable development of disaster mental health services by federal, state, and local agencies, as well as by the American Red Cross and other nonprofit entities. Disaster mental health services are now often provided via on-site crisis intervention and immediate post-impact interventions such as defusing, debriefing, community education, and survivor advocacy (American National Red Cross, 1995; Myers, 1994; Young, Ford, Ruzek,

Friedman, & Gusman, 1998). Such services are preventive in nature and are intended to address normal responses to abnormal situations. They are not generally designed to treat symptoms of post-traumatic stress once they have developed into an established disorder. Despite receiving such preventive interventions, some survivors develop PTSD, and, of course, many of those exposed to disaster do not receive any intervention services. The practical tasks of recovery that require attention during the first weeks and months following disaster may also delay entry into treatment for many individuals who continue to experience high levels of distress. Moreover, many disaster victims do not seek mental health services despite having severe PTSD symptoms. For example, Young, Drescher, Kim-Goh, Suh, & Blake (1998) studied a sample of Korean-Americans following the 1992 Los Angeles Riot and found that the majority of individuals with diagnosable PTSD did not seek treatment (93% and 74% at the 4-month and 16-month intervals, respectively).

In sum, there may remain a significant treatment need among survivors after on-site crisis intervention and immediate post-impact interventions have been delivered. To meet these needs, states may apply for federally-funded crisis-counseling services for disaster victims.[1] Preliminary evidence with other types of trauma survivors indicates that relatively brief therapeutic intervention may reduce the chronicity of subsequent PTSD (Foa, Hearst-Ikeda, & Perry, 1995; Foa, Rothbaum, Riggs, & Murdock, 1991). Therefore, this chapter is an approach to providing time-limited integrative group treatment for disaster survivors who have developed PTSD. The chapter is organized into four sections. The first section outlines treatment objectives. The second presents the rationale for the procedural components selected in this treatment model. The third describes the procedures used, and the final section presents an outline of the 15 sessions of treatment.

GROUP TREATMENT FOR DISASTER-RELATED PTSD: OBJECTIVES

The primary objectives of a time-limited group treatment for disaster survivors are to:

---

[1]Governors of affected states may request a presidential declaration that federal assistance is needed to save lives and protect public health, safety, and property. Following such declarations, state departments of mental health are eligible to apply for funding through the Federal Emergency Management Agency's Immediate Service and Regular Service grants' crisis-counseling programs. If approved, these programs become survivors' primary resource for receiving disaster mental health services. The general objectives of the programs include restoring psychological and social functioning of individuals and the community, while limiting negative mental health outcomes associated with disasters (e.g., PTSD, depression, and substance abuse). The 15-session treatment described here can be delivered within the 9- to 15-month time of the crisis counseling programs.

- Screen prospective participants to specifically target diagnosed Acute Stress Disorder (ASD) or PTSD;

- Refer less severely symptomatic individuals for debriefing or education;

- Refer those diagnosed with other psychiatric problems to appropriate services;

- Reduce the frequency and severity of stress-related symptoms;

- Enhance survivors' control of symptoms of ASD or PTSD;

- Enhance problem-solving to address continuing disaster-related problems.

Treatment Components: Rationale

Most treatment approaches for PTSD include the remembering, describing, and cognitive-emotional integration of traumatic events, and the management of PTSD-related symptoms. In the model described here, several active ingredients of cognitive behavioral therapy for PTSD—trauma-scene identification, direct therapeutic exposure, cognitive restructuring, and self-management skills training—are integrated into a group treatment format. The rationale for each of these components and format is given below.

Group Treatment   There are several potential benefits of treating disaster survivors in a group setting. First, many persons with PTSD believe they are alone in their experiences, and meeting and sharing stories with other survivors can reduce their feelings of isolation. Second, social support is an important aspect of coping with disaster, and a group provides a practical setting in which to ask for and give mutual support. Third, many individuals are reluctant to disclose details of their experience and reactions to it—a reluctance which may interfere with natural recovery processes. The group is a potentially useful vehicle for encouraging such disclosure through modeling. Finally, a group provides a helpful way for participants to learn about coping from other survivors dealing with often similar situations. Potential difficulties with the group format include the challenge to therapists to provide the right balance between the needs of individual members and the needs of the group as a whole, and the challenge of managing the emotional arousal of multiple participants at the same time. In order to facilitate these groups effectively, leaders require two sets of expertise and experience; background in trauma assessment and individual treatment for PTSD and in structured group work. It should be noted that, in some treatment settings, it may not be feasible to assemble suitable numbers of homogeneous disaster survivors to form a group, and that the approach described here may be modified and delivered in the context of individual treatment.

Direct Therapeutic Exposure   From a cognitive-behavioral perspective, direct therapeutic exposure to significant elements of traumatic memories is necessary to reduce trauma-related fears and attain reduction of autonomic responses to related cues or reminders. It is especially important as a way of addressing aspects of PTSD symptomatology (e.g., hyperarousal, reexperiencing symptoms) which, elicited by trauma cues through classical conditioning, may be otherwise unresponsive to voluntary control. According to learning theory, fear reduction is accomplished in part via a process of extinction of fear stimuli through repeated exposure in the absence of aversive stimuli (Barlow, 1988).

The exposure process is also helpful in enabling participants to improve their ability to manage PTSD symptoms. Lyons (1991) noted that "individuals most likely to show long-term positive adjustment may be those who are able to reexperience their trauma with a relatively high degree of voluntary control, either on their own or with the aid of therapy, and who are willing to endure the discomfort of doing so" (p. 98). Horowitz (1993) suggested that trauma survivors who experience intense emotions gradually come to know "that these peaks will be followed by a reduction in intensity, making it possible to 'live through them'" (p. 53).

Direct therapeutic exposure is often an intense emotional experience and participants must be prepared accordingly. Preparation takes place both in pregroup orientation and screening sessions (on a one-to-one basis, often with one of the group leaders), as well as in the first group sessions (sessions one and two in this 15-session model). Preparation involves describing the exposure process and the participant's role in a manner that encourages optimistic but realistic expectancies about both the process and outcome of the procedure. Participants can also be helped to articulate their fears or reservations and encouraged to become actively involved in determining the timing, pacing, content, and intensity of exposure. Preparatory sessions also include a review of coping skills for managing symptoms and seeking social support. Direct therapeutic exposure should be delivered as part of a series of therapeutic interventions that proceeds from preparatory steps (including trauma education and stress management training) through the exposure work to relapse prevention (Keane, 1995).

Exposure may provide a means to reduce fear (and autonomic arousal) associated with trauma experiences, but of equal importance is its role as a platform for participants to process more complex thoughts and emotions that may perpetuate or exacerbate the core traumatic fear reaction. Through therapist-guided exposure, participants can be helped to reexamine their interpretations and conclusions about various aspects of the disaster experience, including issues related to hopelessness, helplessness, guilt, shame, grief, and rage.

Whether the hypothesized mechanism of change is habituation to traumatic stimuli, improvement in ability to cope with strong negative emotions, disconfirmation of trauma-related fears, or restructuring of distressing meanings, repeated exposure will usually be required to facilitate change. In the treatment outlined here, the major tool for ensuring repeated exposure is use of a "Self-Exposure Task" (Appendix 1), i.e., having participants listen several times (two to three times a week) to a tape recording of their trauma narrative.

Cognitive Restructuring   Each individual exposed to trauma will likely experience a variety of distress-producing cognitions related to the event(s) which continue to cause significant levels of distress. For example, Horowitz (1981) analyzed the thematic content of intrusive thoughts and feelings in victims of personal injury and found that discomfort over vulnerability, rage at the source of injury, guilt over responsibility, fear of repetition, and discomfort over aggressive impulses were each present in over 50% of cases, while survivor guilt, sadness over loss, fear of similarity to the victim, rage at those exempted, and fear of loss of control over aggressive impulses were also common. In a discussion of the "coping narratives" of trauma survivors, Meichenbaum and Fitzpatrick (1993) proposed that

> persons who have problems adjusting to negative life events are likely to:
>
> - make unfavorable comparisons between life as it is and as it might have been had the distressing event not occurred;
>
> - engage in comparisons between aspects of life after the stressful event, versus how it was before, and continually pine for what was lost;
>
> - see themselves as victims, with little expectation or hope that things will change or improve;
>
> - blame others for distress and fail to take on any personal responsibility;
>
> - fail to find any meaning or significance in the stressful event;
>
> - dwell on the negative implications of the stressful event;
>
> - see themselves as continually at risk or vulnerable to future stressful events;
>
> - feel unable to control the symptoms of distress (i.e., viewing intrusive images, nightmares, ruminations, psychic numbing, avoidance behaviors, hyperarousal, and exaggerated startle reactions as being uncontrollable and unpredictable);
>
> - remain vigilant to threats and obstacles. (p. 711)

Thoughts about PTSD symptoms may also be important to the etiology, main-tenance, and treatment of PTSD. As Cioffi (1991) suggested in her discussion of somatic interpretation, people can be seen as "active self-diagnosticians" who "act on their internal representations of their illness and of their symptoms; that is, they respond to their private, subjective, sometimes idiosyncratic world of interre-lated beliefs, fears, competencies, and goals" (p. 26). In line with such thinking, Meichenbaum and Fitzpatrick (1993) assert that "it is what survivors say to them-selves and others about their intrusive thoughts, ruminations, and nightmares that figures most prominently in the adjustment process" (p. 711). For example, the disaster survivor whose intrusive images trigger a process of questioning of reli-gious beliefs will have more problems than one who sees such symptoms in more benign terms, or, as Horowitz (1986) noted with regard to the intrusive images which may follow upon trauma, "these frightening experiences may lead to antici-patory anxiety about their recurrence or to secondary anxiety if the subject inter-prets the phenomenon as a sign of losing control or 'going crazy'" (p. 25).

Various authors have noted that it is especially important to process trauma-related information that is incompatible or inconsistent with existing beliefs. Tait and Silver (1989) contend "aspects of the existing system must be altered to accommodate the information, or the event must be reinterpreted in terms that are more assimilable" (p. 366). Roth and Cohen (1986) suggested that the violation of particular pre-trauma beliefs is especially likely to require extensive processing: there are schemata or principles that people have that prevent the uncomplicated assimilation of threatening material. This set of principles includes such basic concepts as: "I do not do bad things; I am intact and invulnerable; there is a just world; my world has meaning and coherence; and I am in control of my life" (p. 815). This same view is found in writers who focus on the "positive illusions" (Taylor, 1989) and "core assumptions" (Janoff-Bulman, 1992) challenged by trau-matic events.

In outlining a theory of cognitive adaptation to threatening events, Taylor (1983) identified three major themes which are central to the cognitive readjust-ment process: "a search for meaning in the experience; an attempt to regain mas-tery over the event in particular and over one's life more generally; an effort to enhance one's self-esteem—to feel good about oneself again despite the personal setback" (p. 1161). Lifton (1979) described similar themes central to the major readjustment tasks of survivors: the need to reestablish a sense of belonging; the need to establish a sense of meaning to the event(s); the need to develop an orientation to the future.

Although each disaster survivor will be troubled by his or her own idiosyn-cratic negative thoughts, commonly held concerns addressed in the treatment approach are described here. These include thoughts and beliefs related to help-lessness and fear, guilt (including survivor guilt), negative self-appraisal, anger and rage at others (including organizations), loss, and ongoing/future implications of the disaster and PTSD symptoms.

- **Helplessness and fear**. Symptoms related to helplessness and fear are likely to be relatively "noncognitive"; that is they may be triggered by exposure to trauma reminders more or less automatically prior to conscious reflection. Fear may be understood as a result of classical conditioning, and as such, may not be under voluntary control and amenable to cognitive interventions. However, people also cognize about their feelings of helplessness and fear. They may consciously conclude, "It is dangerous to experience fear," or "I am helpless to protect myself should another disaster occur." These beliefs, in and of themselves, can add to the distress of survivors, and interfere with adaptive efforts at coping.

- **Guilt**. Beliefs related to guilt, self-blame, and shame are common in the aftermath of trauma and have been correlated with PTSD symptom severity (Kubany & Manke, 1995). When deaths have occurred, "survivor guilt" is common ("I should have died, and they should have lived"). Such beliefs may be especially distressing when survivors attribute the cause of a tragedy to something they did or did not do.

- **Negative self-appraisal**. Much of disaster-related cognition is concerned with the self. Horowitz (1993), for example, noted that "schemas that organize stressful information by the view that the self is bad, damaged, worthless, or incompetent" impede adaptive responding to stressful life events (p. 57). Trauma survivors often believe themselves to have failed, to be weak, or unworthy. Such negative self-appraisal may cause distress, depressed mood, social anxiety and isolation, or maladaptive coping.

- **Anger and rage**. Post-trauma thoughts may also focus on others: Other survivors, community members, rescue workers, organizations and authorities. Did others act appropriately? Were others responsible for the disaster or for some of its effects? What does the experience suggest about others in general, their trustworthiness, motivation, dangerousness? Such thoughts are clinically significant in that they can influence survivors' utilization of social support, their willingness to disclose disaster experiences, and their relationships in general.

- **Loss and ongoing/future implications of the disaster**. Obviously, many survivors suffer loss during and after disaster, including loss of family and friends, possessions or financial resources or both, home and community, jobs and personal roles, health, sense of safety and confidence in the future. Such losses place survivors at risk for chronic bereavement and psychosocial impairment. How do survivors make sense of their loss and their implications for the future? Thoughts regarding the implications of trauma are likely to be clinically important in recovery. Those who undergo traumatic disaster experiences are concerned with the loss of present and future interpersonal relationships, personal capacities, possessions, and access to rewarding activities (e.g., jobs, recreation). These actual and anticipated losses are likely to be the foci of much of the cognitive content processed by individuals as they attempt to come to terms with the event.

Self-Management Skills Training   Helping individuals develop self-management skills to cope with the cardinal symptoms of PTSD (i.e., reexperiencing, behavioral avoidance/psychic numbing, and increased physiological arousal) is central to any treatment of PTSD. In the approach used here, relaxation skills training, attentional focus training, and active problem-focused coping are taught.

• **Relaxation skills training**. Relaxation training is a widely employed component of behavioral treatment for anxiety disorders. Several mechanisms of action have been posited to explain the beneficial effects of relaxation including decreased physiological arousal, reduced generalized anxiety, and improved information processing (Borkovec & Hu, 1990; Borkovec, Lyonfields, Wiser, & Deihl, 1993; Borkovec & Mathews, 1988; Clark, 1994).

Research on relaxation training in the treatment of PTSD has examined the relative effectiveness of various relaxation modalities such as muscle relaxation, deep breathing, thermal biofeedback (Watson, Tuorila, Vickers, Gearhart, & Mendez, 1997); use of relaxation as an adjunctive treatment component (Foa, Hearst-Ikeda, & Perry, 1995; Resick, Jordan, Girelli, Hulter, & Marhoefer-Dvorak, 1988; Silver, Brookes, & Obenchain, 1995); and its impact compared with other primary therapies, e.g., relaxation versus exposure + cognitive restructuring (Echeburua, De Corral, Zubizarreta, & Sarasua, 1997), relaxation versus cognitive restructuring + coping skills training (Echeburua, De Corral, Sarasua, & Zubizarreta, 1996), relaxation versus imaginal exposure and eye movement desensitization (Vaughn et al., 1994). The effects of relaxation have been positive. However, the various relaxation modalities appear to have limited therapeutic value when used alone and are perhaps best utilized in combination with other interventions.

Though reports of adverse affects associated with relaxation are rare, some individuals may experience an intolerable level of transient anxiety practicing relaxation (Borkovec & Heidi, 1980), and there has been a case report of dissociation induced by relaxation training in a combat veteran (Fitzgerald & Gonzalez, 1994). Assessing past adverse reactions to relaxation (imagery/hypnosis) interventions and tailoring the specific relaxation training approach to maximize each participant's sense of self-control are useful precautions.

• **Attentional focus training**. Experiential (Gendlin, 1996; Young, 1990), meditative (Vigne, 1997), and cognitive behavioral (Teasdale, Segal, Williams, & Mark, 1995) approaches to psychotherapy share an emphasis upon focused attention as a means of self-management. Attentional focusing involves shifting attention away from a preoccupation with global negative preoccupations (e.g., worry, self-doubt) to a specific focus on immediate bodily sensations, thoughts (positive affirmations), and feeling states. Consistent with this approach, social psychological and personality research indicates that mindfulness is associated with health (Langer, 1992), while self-consciousness (Saboonchi & Lundh, 1997) and thought suppression (Paulhus & Reid, 1991; Taylor & Brown, 1988; Wenzlaff, Wegner, &

Roper, 1988) are associated with a paradoxical increase in psychophysiologic problems and distress. In the present treatment, relaxation skills training, therapeutic exposure, and cognitive restructuring are all used as opportunities for practicing and reinforcement of attentional focusing skills.

- **Active problem-focused coping**. Research on coping processes has differentiated problem-focused and emotion-focused coping (Folkman & Lazarus, 1980). Coping responses which focus on problem-solving function to remedy the problem itself, while emotion-focused efforts attempt to lessen the negative emotions associated with the problem situation. Several studies with trauma survivors suggest that problem-focused coping is associated with better post-trauma outcomes (Nezu & Carnevale, 1987; Solomon, Mikulincer, & Avitzur, 1988; Solomon, Mikulincer, & Flum, 1988; Wolfe, Keane, Kaloupek, Mora, & Wine, 1993).

Facilitating active and self-enhancing coping can be accomplished by teaching a method of systematic problem-solving (D'Zurilla & Goldfried, 1971). Five steps of problem-solving can be applied to specific current psychosocial dilemmas troubling group participants: Problem definition, brainstorming, solution formulation, experimentation, and evaluation and return to further redefine the problem. This approach can stimulate group discussion about coping options and help participants learn from one another.

COGNITIVE-BEHAVIORAL GROUP TREATMENT FOR DISASTER-RELATED PTSD: 15-SESSION GROUP TREATMENT OUTLINE

Group Design and Session Sequence

We recommend that groups be composed of five to six members and led by two group leaders. Sessions require two hours and take place according to the schedule in the following outline:

Session 1. Introductions, Structure, and Group Rules/Disaster Experience: Similarities and Differences

Objectives

- Introduce group members.

- Explain check-in and check-out processes.

- Explain group goals, structure, and rules.

- Present rationale for group design and explain recovery process.

- Identify and examine members' expectations about recovery.

- Explore and acknowledge differences in disaster experiences.

Presentation/Procedures

1. Explain check-in process and conduct check-in.

2. Orient members to remaining components of Session 1.

3. Describe group structure.

4. Explain group rules.

5. Brief assessments of disaster experience.

6. Discuss similarities and differences in disaster experience.

7. Explain check-out process and conduct check-out.

Session 2. PTSD Education/Self-Management Skills Training

Objectives

- Provide basic PTSD information.

- Provide rationale for learning and using numerous coping strategies to manage PTSD symptoms during and after the group.

- Teach relaxation/attentional skills development and use of relaxation log.

Presentation/Procedures

1. Check-in.

2. Provide basic information about PTSD.

3. Discuss coping with PTSD and trauma-related emotions.

4. Self-management skills training: overview of coping strategies; relaxation and attentional focus training.

5. Check-out.

Session 3. Trauma Scene Identification

Objectives

- Identify coping strategies to be used to control or manage PTSD symptoms during and after the group.

- Help members practice self-management skills (relaxation and attentional focus).

- Identify and reduce fears regarding emotional and social consequences of disclosure.

- Review rationale for tape recording of trauma narrative and self-exposure task.

- Identify trauma scenes to be used during exposure sessions.

Presentation/Procedures

1. Check-in.

2. Self-management skills training: relaxation and attentional focus training.

3. Trauma Scene Identification.

4. Check-out.

Sessions 4–7. Disaster Trauma Memory Exposure (Direct Therapeutic Exposure)

Objectives

- Identify coping strategies to be used to control or manage PTSD symptoms during and after the group.

- Help members practice coping skills (relaxation and attentional focus).

- Ensure structured exposure to important trauma-related stimuli and memories, and prevent cognitive avoidance.

- Discuss emotional and cognitive reactions to the traumatic stories.

- Enhance perceived ability to cope with strong emotional experience.

Presentation/Procedures

1. Check-in.

2. Coping skills training: relaxation and attentional focus training.

1. Direct-therapeutic exposure.

2. Check-out.

Sessions 8–11. Negative Disaster–Related Thoughts (Cognitive Restructuring)

Objectives

- Identify coping strategies to be used to control or manage PTSD symptoms during and after the group.

- Help members practice coping skills (relaxation and attentional focus).

- Prompt discussion and analysis of distressing interpretations of the disaster experiences of members.

- Discuss alternative perspectives on their experiences.

- Distribute and review "Self-Talk Assignment and Affirmation Worksheet."

Presentation/Procedures

1. Check-in.

2. Self-management skills training: relaxation, attentional focus training (affirmation technique).

3. Present cognitive-restructuring sessions.

4. Check-out.

Session 12. Self-Management Skills Training: Affirmation Technique

Objectives

- Identify coping strategies to be used to control or manage PTSD symptoms during and after the group.

- Help members with final development of propositional phrase/affirmation.

- Help members choose markers for behavioral change.

- Teach members how to experience self talk, phrase/affirmation technique while in a state of relaxation.

- Discuss home practice of affirmation technique.

Presentation/Procedures

1. Check-in.

2. Self-management skills training: relaxation, attentional focus training (affirmation technique).

3. Check-out.

Sessions 13–14. Self-Management Skills Training: Problem-Solving about Continuing Disaster-Related Problems

Objectives

- Identify coping strategies to be used to control or manage PTSD symptoms during and after the group.

- Help members practice affirmation technique.

- Emphasize importance of active coping with disaster-related problems.

- Identify current disaster-related problems and help individuals anticipate future problems (e.g., anniversary reactions, reactions to similar weather conditions, holiday gatherings, etc.).

- Use group problem-solving to generate lists of ways of coping with ongoing disaster-related concerns.

- Prompt active coping efforts.

Presentation/Procedures

1. Check-in.

2. Self-management skills training: relaxation, attentional focus training (affirmation technique).

3. Present rationale for session.

4. Discuss ongoing disaster-related problems.

5. Use group problem-solving to generate lists of possible coping actions.

6. Choose coping actions for implementation.

7. Check-out.

Session 15. Summarization and Goodbyes

Objectives

- Discuss lessons learned and implications for the future.

- Identify and discuss feelings about group termination.

Presentation/Procedures

1. Check-in.

2. Presentation of rationale for current session.

3. Group member summarization of key lessons.

4. Discuss group ending.

5. Check-out.

DESCRIPTION OF PROCEDURES

Screening and Selection

A thorough individual screening of prospective group participants is necessary to ensure that individuals are appropriate for group membership. First, it is important to establish a diagnosis of PTSD to ensure that persons with more transient or less severe stress reactions receive less intensive assistance.

Second, it is important to perform a comprehensive assessment of treatment needs, so that problems outside the purview of this group treatment can be addressed. For example, disaster survivors seeking treatment may have been previously exposed to other traumatic events. In cases of traumatic reactivation, assessment necessarily requires differentiating between complicated and uncomplicated PTSD, and correspondingly, matching treatment needs with appropriate treatment modalities (Young, 1992). Also, some candidates for participation may be experiencing a variety of event-precipitated problems, including not only PTSD, but substance abuse, anger, depression, marital or family disturbance, and so on (Green et al., 1992). These problems may occur singly, but more often exist in combination. A broad assessment is therefore required to guide treatment selection, and a range of treatment modalities and procedures may be appropriate to the individual case (e.g., individual or group therapy, medications, anxiety management, couples or family therapy). Concurrent problems may suggest that group exposure treatment, even for those with established PTSD, will be contraindicated (Herman, 1992; Wahlberg, 1997). A medical examination is also recommended because the group work often elicits physiological arousal which may be inadvisable for prospective members with certain health problems (e.g., cardiac disorders).

Third, it is important to include individuals who have had broadly similar disaster experiences. For example, if group members have experienced only property losses, it is unlikely to be beneficial to include a person who has lost members of his or her family in the event. Moreover, the group described herein is not designed to be the primary or sole therapy for individuals who may benefit from family bereavement work (Shapiro, 1994) or who are in need of treatment for complicated mourning (Rando, 1993). Also, since there is relatively little time for cohesion building in this time-limited group, similarity of disaster experience can hasten group cohesion.

Finally, it is essential during the assessment and selection process to orient prospective participants to the group's rationale, structure, procedures, and objectives. Specifically, they should be informed that treatment will involve direct, possibly distressing, discussion of their traumatic experiences. This orientation can increase motivation to attend the group, minimize dropout, and help prepare members for treatment.

Introductions, Structure, and Group Rules: Procedures

The first session is designed to introduce members to one another and review the components, procedures, and rules of the group. The first group is structured as follows:

1. Explain check-in process and conduct check-in.

2. Orient members to remaining components of Session 1.

3. Describe group structure.

   Leaders introduce themselves and describe the design of the group: length, session content and sequencing, etc.

4. Explain group rules.

   Outline, explain, and answer questions about group rules.

   • Confidentiality: Members agree not to disclose the contents of discussion outside the confines of the group; therapists define limits to therapist confidentiality.

   • Showing of mutual respect among members of the group.

   • No pagers, cellphones, candy, food, or smoking.

   • No leaving the room (no bathroom breaks), unless break specified by group leaders.

5. Brief assessments of disaster experience.

   Leaders conduct a person-by-person structured brief assessment of the disaster experience of each member. Ask the following questions of each member: *"Where were you during the disaster?" "What happened to you that was painful or frightening?"*

6. Discuss similarities and differences in disaster experience.

   After restating the importance of communication of mutual respect and the avoidance of minimization of each other's disaster experience, leaders conduct a group discussion to explore similarities and differences in experience. Ask each participant the following: *"In what ways do you see your experiences as being similar to one another? And how about differences? How do you feel different, or what differences do you see between different persons' experiences?"*

7. Explain check-out process and conduct check-out.

The "Check-In/Check-Out" Process

An important component of each session is the check-in/check-out process. Sessions are structured to begin with a check-in process, proceed to the session's topic, and close with a check-out on the part of each member. The systematic process of checking-in provides group leaders with an opportunity to:

- Assess immediate emotional state of participants;

- Review coping efforts since last session;

- Identify issues which need attention prior to other therapeutic activities; and

- Repeat key therapeutic messages.

Similarly, a formal check-out provides one important means to:

- Encourage active participation by all group members;

- Individualize therapeutic learning; and

- Plan for between-session coping and support.

The check-in and check-out processes each require 10 to 20 minutes. Through check-in, each member is given an opportunity to say how he or she is doing, to describe his or her immediate ability to focus on treatment, and to discuss any issues which may cause distraction during the session.

Group members will often describe their current feelings, problems, or reactions to the previous session. To prompt appropriate reporting, leaders can give examples, e.g., highlighting exacerbation of PTSD symptoms such as depression, anger, or urges to drink or use drugs, as well as examples of effective coping. Members should be asked routinely to report on their efforts to cope with their emotions and problems between sessions. When the check-in process is first conducted, it is important that group members are given an explanation of its purpose and procedure—its rationale. This rationale must be described and then discussed with the group in the first session, and regularly repeated and summarized throughout the lifespan of the group. Through this process, members can learn how to make quick and effective use of the check-in routine.

A sample rationale might be:

"We're going to begin each session with a brief check-in so that you can tell us what's going on for you right now, how you're feeling at the moment, and your readiness to be in group today. Everybody brings something with them to group, and the check-in is a time when you can let us know what's on your mind so you can get feedback or help if you need it and so that you can begin to put aside other concerns to concentrate on what's going on here."

"A goal of treatment is to assist you in coping with your worries and emotions so that they don't interfere with your day-to-day functioning. This check-in process is one way of helping you learn to do that."

Following each session's topic, leaders conduct a check-out to end the session. Group members are helped to articulate what they learned about themselves in the session, and to make connections to their own trauma or life experiences. The process is also used to teach participants what to observe in themselves and to take responsibility for asking for support from others (as well as for giving support to others). Members might, for example, be asked: *"What feelings were brought up today?" "What can you do to care for yourselves between sessions?"*

Often, one or more participants will be upset at time of check-out, or concerned with particular issues. When necessary, leaders have the option of planning a coping intervention with these individuals, e.g., *"What can you do tonight, what can we do to help?"*

Coping, symptom management, and support plans can be arranged with input from group members, and group support can be mobilized. Other possibilities, including setting up verbal contracts or utilizing additional mental health services, can be considered. It is important that in the next session's check-in, group leaders follow up with the participant(s) usage of coping plans and the results obtained.

In sum, the check-in, check-out process and coping interventions are used to reinforce the alteration of automatic thoughts, emotional reactions, and impulsive behaviors by inviting members to think through first reactions and their consequences. Through the process of check-in and check-out, members are taught to self-monitor, use active coping, and take responsibility for using support.

PTSD Education   Group members need to learn what constitutes PTSD and have realistic expectations regarding their recovery. In this session, group leaders give an overview of current perspectives on PTSD including the definition of traumatic stress, PTSD symptoms, factors associated with adaptation to disaster, forms of treatment, and treatment outcome.

Information about PTSD is important because it helps members to understand their symptoms and their reactions to the group. Group leaders should explore members' expectations of treatment outcome and the recovery process. Members should be prepared for possible short-term exacerbation of their PTSD symptoms during the group. Anticipatory guidance and help with coping strategies for symptom management provide reassuring therapeutic structure and safety to group members.

Coping with PTSD   This topic extends the PTSD education discussion with a focus on how to increase and broaden the repertoire of participants' coping skills. A list of coping strategies (Appendix 2) is reviewed in the context of managing PTSD symptoms. Group leaders facilitate a discussion, asking participants to identify coping strategies they've used successfully in the past, as well as new strategies they are willing to try. Encouragement can be given to participants to partner-up with other members (for some coping activities, e.g., exercising, recreational activities) to increase and reinforce the benefits of social support. In addition, the first of several discussions about how negative thoughts about PTSD symptoms may impede recovery is undertaken. Participants are given Record of Coping forms (Appendix 3) to monitor symptoms, situations, negative thoughts, and coping efforts between sessions. During each session's Check-in process, members should use their completed Record of Coping forms to guide their report of coping attempts.

Self-Management Skills Training: Relaxation and Attentional Focus Skills Training   Two methods of relaxation, progressive muscle relaxation (Bernstein & Borkovec, 1973) and conscious deep breathing (Young, 1990) are taught. Both procedures include a subset of instructions designed to facilitate attentional focus skills development. For example, during the progressive muscle relaxation procedure, in addition to the conventional instruction to focus attention on the experience of tension or relaxation in a specific muscle group, participants are explicitly instructed to re-focus attention on these physical sensations when they become aware that their attention has shifted. Consequently, participants practice how to focus and refocus their attention. The first self-management skills training session is structured as follows:

1.   Present rationale for learning several strategies for coping with PTSD related symptoms. A sample rationale might be:

> *"As we previously discussed, PTSD affects many aspects of your life and requires more than one stress management strategy to cope with its various symptoms. After each session's check-in, we will devote 15 to 20 minutes to learning and practicing different coping strategies and skills that can be applied to managing your PTSD-related symptoms. In addi-*

tion, we will give you homework assignments to complete between sessions to build upon the coping skills you are learning here or perhaps already use."

2. Give rationale for techniques. A sample rationale might be:

"For the remainder of today's session, we would like for you to begin learning how to experience relaxation while increasing your ability to focus your attention. In later sessions you will learn how to combine and apply these skills to develop positive thoughts that counter negative thinking. We also examine several other problem-solving and stress management strategies."

"A common component of many PTSD treatments is teaching various relaxation techniques. One helpful and easy-to-learn technique is progressive muscle relaxation. We modify it slightly to show you how to focus and refocus your attention. Eventually, you will learn how to apply the skill of attentional focus on positive thoughts while in a state of relaxation."

3. Discuss technique and overview of process. A sample introduction and overview might be:

"Today, we will begin with the modified muscle relaxation technique. For the next two sessions, you will learn and practice this technique here and at home. Three weeks from today, we will learn a conscious deep breathing technique that also induces relaxation and helps develop your ability to focus your attention. You will have to practice these techniques daily between our sessions to learn them quickly. We will give you handouts [leaders must prepare a handout describing procedure; use description presented below as a template] *and a log* ["Relaxation Log," Appendix 4] *for monitoring whether or not these techniques are helping you to experience relaxation. In future sessions we will have more in-depth discussions about disaster-related thoughts and you will receive a written assignment to complete* ["Self-Talk Affirmation Technique Worksheet," Appendix 5]. *This assignment builds on the work done in the session and will help you identify negative disaster thoughts and alternative positive thoughts or self-talk. In our last few sessions together, we will practice how to combine relaxation, focused attention, and self-talk to increase your ability to counter negative disaster-related thoughts."*

"Before we begin, we would like you to fill out a log that records your current level of tension/relaxation, so that we have it to compare to your level after the relaxation procedure and after several weeks of training. Please fill out this log daily, before and after you practice the relaxation procedures at home."

4. Facilitate modified progressive muscle relaxation procedure. A sample instruction narrative might be:

"The progressive muscle relaxation procedure is simple. With my guidance you will carefully tighten and relax various muscle groups in your body. As you tighten the muscle group, please focus your entire attention on the experience of tension in those muscles. Make the sensation the entire focus of your attention. As you relax, again focus all your attention on the sensations you experience in that muscle group. You can expect that your attention will shift. This is natural. When you become aware that your attention has shifted, use this as a signal to remind you to refocus on the current muscle group. Avoid any criticism of yourself when you have noticed that your attention has shifted. The key is to bring your attention back each time you notice it has shifted without any additional interference. I will periodically remind you to refocus your attention. Please sit comfortably, but not in a position that is likely to cause you to fall asleep, and adjust your clothing and take off eyeglasses, as we prepare to start. Any questions?"

"Let's begin. Starting with your head and working your way down to your feet, observe any sensations you have in your body. Simply observe where your body is holding tension and where it is relaxed. Write down on the relaxation log, using the triangle to indicate "before"—the corresponding level of relaxation or tension that you feel. Now lets begin with the first step. You may wish to close your eyes, but if you feel uncomfortable doing so, find a spot in front of you to look at. As we move through the different muscle groups, do not do anything that might aggravate any medical condition you may have. Simply skip that muscle group."

"Please tighten your right foot (pointing toes away from your body), focusing your entire attention on the experience/sensations of tension in your right foot. Tighten the muscles in your foot hard as you can without causing cramping. Hold the tension. If you begin to think about something else, simply bring your attention back to the sensations in your right foot. Hold the tension for two more seconds."

"Now relax the right foot, paying attention to the change in sensations. Once again, if your mind has wandered, bring it back to the sensations in your right foot without any self-criticism or other thought. Repeat tightening your right foot."

Leader continues with the protocol outlined below, periodically reminding members to refocus their attention. Each muscle contraction (tension) is completed in approximately three to four seconds. Each release of the contraction (relaxation) is completed in five to six seconds. The instruction narrative continues as follows:

- *Tighten right calf (straighten leg and point toes toward your body). Relax. Repeat.*

- *Tighten right thigh (straighten leg and contract thigh muscles). Relax. Repeat.*

- *Deep full inhalation, full exhalation.*

- *Tighten left foot (straighten leg and point toes away from your body). Relax. Repeat.*

- *Tighten left calf (straighten leg and point toes toward your body). Relax. Repeat.*

- *Tighten left thigh (straighten leg and contract thigh muscles). Relax. Repeat.*

- *Deep full inhalation, full exhalation.*

- *Tighten buttocks. Relax. Repeat.*

- *Tighten stomach (bring stomach in towards spine). Relax. Repeat.*

- *Tighten chest (squeezing shoulders together). Relax. Repeat.*

- *Deep full inhalation, full exhalation.*

- *Tighten shoulders and neck (raise shoulders toward your ears). Relax. Repeat.*

- *Slowly bring right ear toward right shoulder left ear toward left shoulder chin toward chest, return to normal position. Repeat.*

- *Deep full inhalation, full exhalation.*

- *Tighten jaw. Relax. Repeat.*

- *Tighten nose. Relax. Repeat.*

- *Tighten eyes gently. Relax. Repeat.*

- *Tighten forehead (raise eyebrows toward ceiling). Relax. Repeat.*

- *Deep full inhalation, full exhalation.*

- *Tighten right hand (make fist as if squeezing a rubber ball). Relax. Repeat.*

- *Tighten right forearm (straighten arm, lock elbow, and bend wrist backwards). Relax. Repeat.*

- *Tighten right upper arm (bend elbow, tightening bicep, like you were Popeye). Relax. Repeat.*

- *Deep full inhalation, full exhalation.*

- *Tighten left hand (make fist as if squeezing a rubber ball). Relax. Repeat.*

- *Tighten left forearm (straighten arm, lock elbow, and bend wrist backwards). Relax. Repeat.*

- *Tighten left upper arm (bend elbow, tightening bicep, like you were Popeye). Relax. Repeat.*

- *Deep full inhalation, full exhalation.*

    "Okay, when you feel ready, orient yourself to the room. What was the exercise like for you? Does anyone have any questions? Record on the relaxation log, using the plus sign to indicate "after," the corresponding level of relaxation or tension that you feel. Did anyone's tension increase?"

In subsequent sessions, leaders can collapse muscle groups to abbreviate the procedure (e.g., "tighten feet, lower legs, and thighs simultaneously"), checking to see if members are able to reach significant levels of relaxation with the shortened process. Members are more likely to maintain practice at home if they can learn how to experience relaxation in less time.

The *conscious deep breathing technique* is structured as follows:

1. Review guidelines for technique:

    - Each repetition of inhalation and exhalation is done slowly and quietly (*"Another person should not be able to hear your breathing."*).

    - Each inhalation and exhalation is executed for as long as possible without discomfort while the primary focus of attention is on the sensation of breathing in and out.

    - There are four steps and each step is repeated three times. Members are instructed to keep track of each step and repetition. A useful method of tracking is to begin with the thumb placed on the lowest of the three sections of the index finger. For each repetition, the thumb is moved one section upward. For each successive step, the corresponding successive finger is used until the thumb has reached the top section of the "pinky."

2.   Ask members to record level of relaxation or tension on relaxation log.

3.   Ask members to sit comfortably and close eyes. Members who wish to keep eyes open are asked to focus attention on a spot in front of them. Begin guiding members through the four steps.

   • Inhale through nose. Hold two seconds. Exhale through nose.

     (Thumb on index finger.) Repeat twice.

   • Inhale through nose. Hold two seconds. Exhale through mouth.

     (Thumb on middle finger.) Repeat twice.

   • Inhale through mouth. Hold two seconds. Exhale through nose.

     (Thumb on ring finger.) Repeat twice.

   • Inhale through mouth. Hold two seconds. Exhale through mouth.

     (Thumb on pinky.) Repeat twice.

4.   Ask members to resume their natural form of breathing and to reorient to the room. Inquire about members' experiences and invite questions. Ask members to record level of relaxation or tension on relaxation log. Ask if anyone's level of tension increased.

Self-Talk Affirmation Technique

After the session about negative disaster-related thoughts and counterarguments, a homework assignment, Self-Talk Affirmation Technique Worksheet (Appendix 4), is given in preparation for learning an additional attentional focus modality, referred to as an affirmation technique (Young, 1990). The affirmation technique is an integration of the relaxation, attentional focus, and the cognitive restructuring work previously practiced by group members and is similar to the popular relaxation-response technique described by Benson (1975), with one important modification. Instead of choosing one word, the individual substitutes a propositional phrase (an affirmation) developed from the Self-Talk and Affirmation Technique Worksheet.

   The affirmation technique is designed to teach participants how to focus and refocus their attention on the propositional phrase or affirmation while in a state of deep relaxation. Each phrase or affirmation may be divided into two or three sections. If divided into two sections, the first part of the phrase or affirmation becomes the subject of thought during an extended inhalation. The inhalation is followed by a 2- or 3-second holding of the breath. The second half of the phrase or affirmation is the subject of thought during an extended exhalation. If divided into three sections, the phrase or affirmation is divided to correspond with the inhalation, holding of breath, and exhalation. An example of how to divide a propositional phrase or affirmation to correspond to the cycle of breathing is given below:

Example propositional phrase/affirmation:

"I can control my anger, I can choose how to express it."

Dividing phrase in two sections:

Inhalation	**2-second hold**	**Exhalation**
"I can control my anger"		"I can choose how to express it"

Dividing phrase/affirmation into three sections:

Inhalation	**2-second hold**	**Exhalation**
"I can	control my anger.	I can choose how to express it"

Applying the attentional focus skills learned while practicing the progressive muscle and conscious breathing techniques, members are taught how to practice focusing and refocusing their attention on the phrase. The procedure for the affirmation technique is structured as follows:

1. Group leader facilitates an abbreviated version of the progressive muscle relaxation and conscious breathing procedures.

2. Maintaining the relaxed atmosphere, group leader asks members to begin focusing their attention on their individual phrase while taking in a deep and extended inhalation.

3. Instructions are given to continue focused attention on the affirmation while holding and exhaling the breath. Instructions are repeated several times. Members are then given a few minutes to continue the procedure on their own. Periodically, the group leader reminds members to bring their attention back to their affirmation without any other self talk, e.g., *"Your attention may have wandered, that's okay, simply bring it back to the affirmation and avoid telling yourself 'Oh, my mind wandered, I'm not good at this.'"* The group leader continues to alternate between in-

structing members to repeat the procedure on their own and giving them explicit instructions to refocus. The entire protocol runs for 10 minutes.

Note, that in the course of reviewing the Self-Talk and Affirmation Assignment group leaders will be required to use clinical judgment to evaluate if any of these propositions are an expression of negative or distorted styles of thinking (Burns, 1980), or unrealistic expectations, (e.g., "I shouldn't let things bother me." "I shouldn't be nervous."). Group time can be used to help members modify affirmations so that they represent a realistic or helpful cognitive adaptation (e.g., "When something bothers me, I can help myself." "I can practice and experience relaxation.").

Members are instructed how to practice each of the procedures at home and given handouts as guidelines. Daily home practice is essential to members' acquiring and maintaining the self-management skills of relaxation, attentional focus, and self-talk/affirmation.

Self-Management Skills Training: Active-Problem Focused Coping   Many disaster-related problems (e.g., loss of resources, disaster aid procedures, rebuilding issues) continue long past the initial period of acute recovery and continue to cause distress for the survivor. How the individual copes with these challenges is one influence on long term outcome. So, it is important to encourage active adaptive coping.

Group leader may begin with the following rationale:

> *"During our past meetings, we've focused on your trauma memories and disaster-related thoughts. In this session, we want to focus on the role of active coping. Some problems caused by the disaster are not easily solvable and will continue to challenge your abilities to cope. It is important that you take an active approach to coping."*

> *"You may have had limited responsibility for events due to lack of control over the behavior of others, the stress and confusion of disaster, limited availability of information, and so on. Similarly, you cannot be held responsible and blamed for your emotional reactions to the disaster and your PTSD symptoms. But, you are responsible now for taking action toward recovery from PTSD and toward active coping with problems."*

The group is asked to generate a list of problems caused by the disaster which cause continuing difficulties. Examples include:

- Pain or disability due to injury

- Financial problems

- Unemployment

- Homelessness

- Legal processes

- Problems with disaster relief applications

In sessions 12 and 13, one significant ongoing problem faced by each group member is taken as the topic of discussion, and the group helps identify coping actions. Focusing on one individual at a time, the group helps the individual generate possible coping actions. The person is then helped by the leader, with input from the group, to problem solve in order to identify actions that seem most useful as well as to determine how to begin to implement them prior to next session.

Immediately after the group has identified a list of coping actions for the individual's problem, the member should be asked to select several of the actions for implementation. He or she should be asked to identify which actions will be put into practice and asked to report on the experience at the next session. Each member should complete this problem solving exercise at least once in this two-session block.

Trauma Scene Identification   It is important to acknowledge and address fears of recalling a trauma scene and disclosing the associated details and emotions. The fear of losing emotional control may cause some group members to omit upsetting elements, minimize events, avoid details during the recounting of memories, or use language which distorts their emotions (e.g., "He left us," versus "He was blown apart."). Fear of not being able to stop crying, not receiving support, of going crazy or going off and becoming violent is common. The therapists can speak directly to these concerns and give realistic reassurance regarding them.

Detail and emotionality of trauma stories are also influenced by social factors. Participants may be concerned about the social acceptability of their actions and expect negative responses to them. They may have encountered real or imagined condemnation by those they previously spoke to, or others who may not have wanted to hear their stories. In group, participants could omit or modify details out of fear of pushing others away, or they might not reveal the intensity of their emotions out of a lack of trust or dislike of certain members. Issues related to actual and expected reactions of members, as well as trust and disliking should be discussed.

Trauma scene identification sessions are structured as follows:

1. Provide rationale for recalling trauma scene.

2. Conduct a discussion about fears of thinking about and disclosing details of trauma.

    "Many people who participate in counseling groups are anxious about what will happen if they talk about their traumatic experiences, what will happen with their emotions, and how will other people react to hearing their stories? What concerns each of you about opening yourself up and telling your stories?"

3. Leaders ask questions to prompt discussion of the following common concerns:

    *   Loss of control

    *   Increased emotional pain

    *   Inability to stop crying

    *   Rejection or condemnation by others

    During the discussion, leaders interject information about other potential emotional reactions (e.g., rage, guilt, helplessness) reassuring members of their normalcy and that, although the feelings may be frightening, they can be dealt with in a new manner without negative consequences. Other common reactions members should be prepared to possibly experience and manage include:

    *   Presence of physical symptoms

    *   Amnesia for some past traumatic events

    *   Increased dreaming

    *   Increased thoughts about alcohol/drugs

    *   Reactivation of strong emotions linked to prior traumatic events

4. Leaders review rationale for tape recording of trauma narrative and self-exposure task.

    "We understand it's upsetting to think about disaster experiences, but we know from our work and clinical research that as survivors recount their

experiences, they begin to cope more effectively with their memories and emotions. Part of treatment involves reviewing your experiences enough times so that you feel less fear and pain when doing so. As we discussed in the pregroup meeting, a tape recording of your trauma narrative is made for your use and is an important tool in your recovery. With the aid of the work we do here, frequently listening to the tape will enable you to practice techniques to cope with distressful feelings and thoughts effectively. There are several options for when and how to use the tape. We want you to use the tape when you feel ready to do so. When you feel ready, you can listen to the tape on the day of a group meeting, sometime before session; you can listen alone or in the presence of a trusted friend or family member. The tape remains in your possession and you are in control of using it for this part of your recovery."

5.   Leaders help members to identify disaster-related traumatic scenes.

Direct Therapeutic Exposure   Exposure sessions are conducted one member at a time, with two participants given guided exposure each session. Group leaders meet to select the order in which individuals are to describe their traumatic experiences. Clinical judgment is the basis for these decisions, and criteria for selection can include evaluating participants' current emotional state and their relative ability to model the procedure in terms of providing an emotionally-congruent narrative, demonstrating relatively effective coping skills, and receptivity to suggestion.

Each participant is given one in-session opportunity to describe his or her chosen traumatic disaster experiences. Leaders should generally respect participants' choices, while encouraging them to select emotionally significant experiences. The Self-Exposure Task occurs between sessions, when members are asked to listen several more times (usually 2 to 3 times a week) to the tape recording of their trauma narrative. Group leaders must ensure successful recording of the in-session narrative. To maintain confidentiality, the recorded segment should only include the member's trauma narrative and accompanying therapists' remarks, and not the postnarrative group discussion. The Direct Therapeutic Exposure is structured as follows:

1.   Check-in.

2.   Describe the task.

Tell group members it is their task to talk about their most upsetting or important traumatic experiences during the disaster, including details of what they saw, heard, and experienced, and their thoughts, feelings, and sensations during the experience.

> *"We would like you to describe, in detail, a significant, upsetting disaster-related experience. It's important to use today's time to cover the things most troubling and painful to you, and not avoid telling us about things you feel ashamed, guilty, or embarrassed about. We want to support and help you take the risks of sharing and acknowledging what happened. We want to know what you saw, heard, and felt, and what you were thinking and feeling at the time. I will be guiding you to focus on different parts of the experience and to remember details. Please share as much as you can, but what you share is your choice at all times."*

> *"The most important memories to discuss are ones that continue to cause you distress and interfere with your daily life. These memories may be related to events and experiences that you think about often, or that show up in your dreams. They might have to do with strong emotions like guilt, shame, terror, helplessness, grief, or sadness. They might be related to powerful and disturbing images of things you witnessed or experienced."*

> *"I will also be asking you how you're feeling as you tell your story. We don't want you to be overwhelmed, but we do want you to be able to acknowledge to yourself and the group any painful feelings that arise."*

> *"… (co-therapist) will be following along but will be watching the group as a whole to monitor, and if necessary, respond to other members' reactions to your account. We will attempt to preserve your time so that you don't lose your focus. Consequently, if any one of you listening have a strong reaction, we will most likely ask you to remember it, and bring it up after _____ (narrator) is finished."*

3. Identification of members/selection of disaster experiences.

   Tell the group which members have been selected to tell their disaster stories. Ask the first person to briefly identify the traumatic experience he or she has selected.

   > *"We realize that you may have experienced a number of frightening or upsetting experiences during _____ . Please tell us which particular experience you decided to focus on today, and why you've made that choice."*

4. Begin tape recording.

5. Begin the trauma account.

   The course of the narrative should include details of the experience, the identification of thoughts experienced during and after the trauma, and expression of emotion during the narrative.

*"Okay_____, are you ready to begin? You selected_____
as your first scene, so please begin with telling us what happened and
what your feelings and thoughts were as it was happening."*

Allow the survivor to use his or her own words. When necessary, use
questions to encourage elaboration of statements, seek clarification, or
interpretation of events. Often, survivors have told a version of their
experience several times before having sought treatment. Generally, these
accounts neglect important details. Enrich the context of memory retrieval by selectively asking questions about moment-to-moment details
of places and events.

If the emotional tone of their story is flat, ask questions about feelings to
increase the emotionality of the account. If the narrator becomes silent,
ask:

*"What are you remembering?" "What are you thinking or feeling right
now?"*

Whenever possible, let him or her know why you are asking the question:

*"I saw a look on your face and wondered if you were having some strong
feelings about that."*

As the story unfolds, care should be taken to ensure the narrator does not
avoid important aspects of the experience. To minimize avoidance and
ensure attention to important issues, ask questions about:

*   Bodily/mental reactions (e.g., freezing, shaking, confusion, sense
    that things were not real, sense of seeing events from a distance).

*"What are you feeling in your body right now?" "What are you saying
to yourself right now?"*

*   Feelings of fear, panic, sadness, anger.

*"Can you pay attention to, and stay with, what you're feeling right
now?"*

*   Thoughts and feelings about bodily reactions and emotional
    feelings.

*"What are you saying to yourself about what's happening, or about how
you're feeling?"*

Throughout these sessions, the leader who is not guiding the narrator monitors responses of group members who are hearing the story. It is important to inquire about members who begin crying or appear to be experiencing other strong emotions during the story. Bearing in mind that continuity of narration is important, a clinical judgment is necessary regarding the allotment of time attending to a member who demonstrably reacts. Often, it will suffice to say, for example:

"John, I can see that you had a strong reaction to Jane's experience. Pay attention to what caused you to react strongly so that we can talk about it after Jane is finished."

Members are also monitored for signs of tuning out or dissociation. Those who do so can be brought back to the present by reminding them of the importance of listening to the narrator, conveying your interest in their reaction, and letting them know that after the account is completed, you will be asking them about what happened. In extreme cases, using a warm but firm tone, instruct the individual to look at a timepiece and tell you the time, or verbally orient him or her to the room, date, time, and the safety of the situation, for example:

"Tom, you are sitting here with us in the county building, its Wednesday, July 3, 7:45 p.m., and you're safe here. Repeat to me what I just said."

Return to the narration as soon as possible and upon its completion, ask the member who dissociated:

"Where are you right now?" "Where did you go before?" "Did you have trouble relating to what _____ was saying?"

6. Ask about additional trauma-related themes.

After the disaster event or experience has been described in some detail from start to finish, it will be helpful to briefly ask about other disaster-related themes, if they have not been mentioned earlier.

- Perceived consequences of actions (e.g., others suffered or died).

- Reactions of others (e.g., viewed negatively by others, avoided by them).

- Impact on self-image and self-esteem.

- Sense of betrayal by God, authorities, or others (e.g., random senseless destruction; public relation spins; relief procedure obstacles;

poor leadership; inadequate preparation or information). For example, many migrant victims of the 1985 Mexico City earthquake who later were victimized by 1989 Loma Prieta earthquake, believed they were deservedly being punished by God.

7. Stop tape recording.

8. Ask about reactions to telling about traumatic disaster experiences (do not record).

   Be vigilant for shame, guilt, concern about reactions of other group members, anger, fears about continuing emotional upset and worsened PTSD symptoms. Explore specific negative reactions to disclosure if it seems appropriate.

   "You've just told us about some very painful and upsetting experiences. How do you feel about having gone through all this with us?"

   "During some of our first meetings in this group, we discussed some of the fears that people might have about telling their stories, fears about breaking down emotionally, shame, negative reactions of others, and so on. What concerns do you have about what you've been saying today?"

9. Invite other group members to comment.

   Invite group members to share their feedback and observations with the individual who has described his or her disaster experiences. After their comments, ask them:

   "What did you learn for yourself today?"

10. Ask next member to begin disaster account and begin tape recording (new tape). Repeat process as outlined above.

11. Prepare members to cope between sessions.

    Ask members to anticipate how they will be feeling and reacting immediately following the group and through the following days. Help them develop coping plans for the time between sessions. Focus on members who have recounted their experiences, but attend to needs of other members as well.

    Ask members about coping:

    "How did you deal with what happened immediately following the events?"

"What did you do to cope with your feelings about what had happened?"
"What have you done in the past to cope successfully with difficult situations or problems?"

Ask about the following potential reactions:

• Shutting down

• Isolating /keeping others away

• Alcohol/drug abuse

• Denying importance of the events

• Anger /aggression/retaliation

• Exaggerated sense of responsibility for others

"You've done some difficult things here today. You've described painful memories and identified how you've coped in the past; you've received feedback from each other. As we've discussed before, your PTSD symptoms are likely to be strong now because you have willingly opened yourself to the memories and not avoided all your painful thoughts and feelings.

"Now is the important time for you to work at developing a new style of coping with your memories and symptoms. This will be hard, but it's very important. What are you willing to do to deal with your distress between now and our next meeting?"

"How can we help as a group?"

"What are the other members of the group willing to do to support ... as he/she works toward more positive ways of coping?"

12. Assign self-exposure task.

During exposure sessions, every member of the group will have one opportunity to recount his or her traumatic disaster experience. However, such traumatic exposure should be repeated in order to increase the likelihood of therapeutic benefits. Repetition of exposure is achieved via a self-exposure task.

Once again, leaders present rationale for repeated exposure and facilitate discussion about the self-exposure component of treatment.

"As you know, we've made a tape recording for you to listen to and think about. It will help you digest everything that we talked about. Remember, the tape is intended to serve as a tool in your recovery. By listening to it a number of times, you can begin to learn to effectively manage the feelings and distressing thoughts it brings up. We want you to do this when you feel ready. You are in control of this part of your recovery."

To minimize negative reactions to initial efforts, the survivor should arrange for some form of social support immediately after self-exposure. Remind members of their options for when and how to use the tape:

- Listen to the tape on the day of the next group meeting, in the morning or afternoon before the session.

- Listen to the tape in the presence of a trusted friend or family member who was not a victim of the disaster.

Group leaders identify when and under what conditions the individuals in the group plan to listen to their tape, and explain the Self-Exposure Task Record (Appendix 5).

13. Check-out.

Cognitive Restructuring The accounts of trauma lead therapists to identify negative, distorted interpretations of the events which perpetuate distress and prevent recovery. Questions of culpability, predictability, and controllability of traumatic events are important because inappropriate self- or other-blame may cause intense feelings of guilt and anger that exacerbate distress, depression, and PTSD symptomatology.

Negative beliefs related to disaster experiences sometimes perpetuate distress and may prevent recovery. It is important to address these distressing understandings, and help the survivor find more constructive perspectives on his or her experience. In these sessions, therapists raise core themes (related to common negative disaster-related thoughts) for consideration and discussion within the group. The accounts of trauma generated in earlier sessions will help identify particular beliefs causing distress for specific group members.

Recommended content for Sessions 8 to 11:

Session 8.   Helplessness and fear.

Session 9.   Guilt and thoughts about self.

Session 10.   Anger and rage.

Session 11.   Loss and ongoing/future implications of the disaster and its effects.

To manage effective discussion of these themes, group leaders must anticipate the kinds of negative interpretations and conclusions drawn by members, and develop an effective repertoire of counterarguments or self-statements and beliefs which present alternative, more forgiving interpretations of events. Some common disaster-related negative thoughts and possible counterarguments, grouped by theme, are presented in Table 9.1.

The procedure for cognitive restructuring is as follows:

1.   Present rationale for cognitive-restructuring sessions.

   Give rationale for reviewing some of the attitudes and beliefs about disaster that continue to cause problems, and for the intention of finding ways for members to feel less distress.

   "We've talked a lot about some very traumatic things that happened to you all. Now we want to help you take a look at some of your interpretations about what happened as well as the conclusions that you drew from your experience. Maybe we can help you find some new and less distressing ways to think about what happened."

2.   Outline key disaster theme.

   Outline the current theme and its relationship to disaster-related traumatic experience. Make reference where possible (based on knowledge gained during previous sessions) to examples of the current theme as it applies to members, (e.g., guilt).

   "For example, John, you shared with us in an earlier session that you felt you made the wrong decision by not following evacuation orders which, in turn, resulted in the severe injury of your son. As I understand you, this belief that you are responsible for his injury and cannot be forgiven continues to cause you much distress."

3.   Lead discussion of theme.

   "Today, lets talk about this theme of (guilt) following disaster. What thoughts and feelings do you have about blame and guilt?"

TABLE 9.1 Common Disaster-Related Negative Thoughts and Possible Counterarguments

Theme	Negative Thoughts	Counterarguments
Helplessness & fear.	I was helpless then, and I won't be able to cope with future events either.	I may have felt helpless, but my actions saved my life, and I can continue to help myself.
	It's unacceptable to experience fear like this.	Fear is natural and helped me to survive. Gradually, I can ease out of it.
	The world is an extremely dangerous place and I must be constantly on guard to protect myself.	There are times that I need to be on guard and times that I don't. I don't always have to be on guard.
	My kids will never be safe again.	Everything in reason is/has been done to keep my kids safe.
	My kids will be scarred for life.	Other kids heal from loss and so can mine.
Guilt & thoughts about self.	Because of me, other people died; I should have prevented their deaths.	Many factors beyond my control resulted in the deaths that occurred.
	I was a coward.	I felt afraid, but my actions kept me from further injury.
	I should have helped my neighbor.	Stopping could have caused greater problems.
	I should have had emergency supplies on hand.	The disaster could have destroyed all supplies. I was creative with the supplies I had.
	There's something wrong with me; I should have gotten over this by now.	It takes time and patience to get over this. I'm not the only one going through this.
Anger & rage.	Other people can't be trusted to help.	There are people who can/ will help me, and there are people who can't or won't.

Table 9.1 continues on page 186.

TABLE 9.1 Continued

Theme	Negative Thoughts	Counterarguments
	The authorities are only interested in saving money.	It is difficult to apply for relief, but persistence and building a strong case is my best defense.
	If the inspections were done, this wouldn't have happened.	I feel angry about their negligence and I am going to do what I can to see that it doesn't happen again.
Loss and ongoing/future implications of disaster and PTSD symptoms	I'll never get over this; it'll ruin my life.	People rebuild their lives. Each week I can do something to make my life better.

After acquiring examples of guilt-related thinking, therapists gradually move into the process of helping members challenge their self-blame.

4. Help members challenge or reframe negative beliefs and conclusions.

While acknowledging how painful certain beliefs are, therapists help participants challenge the validity (accuracy and completeness) of some trauma-related conclusions. It is important to use group feedback to provide more positive alternative interpretations of events. This process often naturally produces empathic comments from members as they help one another see things from new perspectives. During the discussion, it is useful if one of the therapists lists counterarguments (e.g., reasons why guilt is unwarranted or exaggerated) on a flip chart or board. Therapists will need to be creative in prompting members to identify alternative perspectives or counterarguments. Therapists can ask leading questions:

"Should you accept sole responsibility for what happened?"

Or, restate the negative belief in exaggerated form:

"You should have been perfect in the way you handled the situation!"

The exaggeration can give attention to parts of the belief that are open to challenge. One way to generate additional counterbeliefs is to ask group members the following questions:

"If this had happened to a friend or family member, what would you say to him?" or "What would you think of her?" or, "If you had been injured instead of him, would you have wanted him to feel guilty about your injury?"

Often, given the conditions under which the disaster occurred, group members could not have predicted or controlled events and therefore cannot reasonably assume blame for their occurrence. Williams (1987) listed several useful ways to help those suffering from survivor guilt to realize they did the best they could under the circumstances:

- Drawing attention to the limited time during which decisions were taken, the amount of experience they had in such decision-making situations, and the amount of information they had at the time;

- Investigating whether others shared some of the responsibility for decisions, by direct action or the approval of action;

- Identifying as many positive aspects as possible of the person's behavior during the trauma.

5. Lead reflection on implications of discussion.

Ask the group, and especially the members most troubled by the theme under discussion, how the considerations generated during the discussion fit with their negative beliefs:

"Looking back on things, several people here have acknowledged that they made a decision which was understandable given what they knew at the time. How does that fit with some of you blaming yourselves for making a bad decision?"

Therapists can summarize parts of the discussion and describe aspects of the disaster experience that don't fit with the belief as it applies to individuals in the group:

"It seems you all agree that your actions were reasonable given your past experience with hurricane warnings? And, that there wasn't a way you could have known that this one would be different. And, that John, had you attempted to evacuate at the time, you and the others might have been injured or killed."

6. Distribute and discuss Self-Talk and Affirmation Assignment.

Summarization and Goodbyes In the final session, leaders help participants to strengthen their new understandings by asking them to identify new
insights, rehearse constructive attitudes, and think about implications for the
future. Because loss and abandonment are trauma-related cues for many trauma
survivors, it is important that group leaders directly address the experience of
group termination for participants. In the last meeting, leaders allot an equal time
for individual review (see description below), and facilitating a group discussion
of group termination. In this way there is a discussion of both subjects during the
final session.

1. Check-in.

2. Presentation of rationale for current session.

    *"The purpose of our last session is to help you identify and summarize
    main lessons learned that can help you cope in the future, and to explore
    how we as a group feel about ending our time together."*

3. Group member summarization of key lessons.

    Ask each member in turn to identify what he or she has learned in the
    group:

    • about ways of coping with stress and PTSD; about disaster
      memories;

    • about ability to deal with those memories and PTSD symptoms;

    • about future coping tools.

    Group discussion centers on these themes.

    *"During our last meeting together, I am going to ask each of you to tell
    us a little about what you have learned about yourself. Especially, about
    how you have been trying to cope, how you plan to cope in the future,
    what obstacles you think might prevent you from continued good coping,
    and what your strategy might be to overcome such obstacles. I'll help
    you know what to tell us by asking questions. _____ , how about
    starting."*

    *"What have been your main negative beliefs related to your disaster
    experiences? How are you going to challenge those beliefs in the
    future?"*

4. Discuss group ending.

Ask members to express their thoughts and feelings about their group experience and about ending the group. Encourage them to take the view that the end of the group is the beginning of their work of learning to cope more effectively with PTSD-related emotions and life problems.

"Our group is going to be ending very soon. Let's talk today about what benefits you received from participating in the group, and what has not happened that you had hoped for. Also, how you feel about the group ending, and saying goodbye to everyone."

5. Check-out.

CONCLUSION

In this chapter, we have presented the rationale, procedures, and detailed session outlines for a cognitive-behavioral group treatment of disaster-related PTSD. It is important to note that this approach has been constructed from clinical experience, and remains to be empirically validated; hence, it should be regarded as a starting point for the development of group treatments for PTSD related to disaster exposure. We present the material because it is our observation that most of the writing and research on disaster mental health has focused on the acute phase of disaster recovery and on early intervention to prevent development of chronic postdisaster problems. Guidelines for treatment of PTSD once it has developed are also important. The approach outlined here adapts methods developed with other groups of trauma survivors, especially combat veterans, and is faithful to the principles and procedures currently employed in cognitive-behavioral treatments of PTSD. Specifically, it incorporates aspects of direct therapeutic exposure, cognitive restructuring, self-management skills training, and active problem-focused coping skills training to address some of the medium-term needs of disaster survivors with PTSD.

REFERENCES

American National Red Cross. (1995). *Disaster mental health services I. Participant's workbook.* Washington, DC: Author.

Barlow, D. H. (1988). *Anxiety and its disorders: The nature and treatment of anxiety and panic.* New York: Guilford Press.

Benson, H. (1975). *The relaxation response.* New York: William Morrow.

Bernstein, D. A. , & Borkovec, T. D. (1973). *Progressive relaxation training: A manual for the helping professions.* Champaign, IL: Research Press.

Bland, S. H., O'Leary, E. S., Farinaro, E., Jossa, F., & Trevisan, M. (1996). Long-term psychological effects of natural disasters. *Psychosomatic Medicine, 58,* 18–24.

Bromet, E. J., Parkinson, D.K., Schulberg, H. C., Dunn, L. O., & Gondek, P.C. (1982). Mental health of residents near the Three Mile Island reactor: A comparative study of selected groups. *Journal of Preventive Psychiatry, 1,* 225–274.

Borkovec, T. D., & Heidi, F. (1980, December). *Relaxation-induced anxiety: Psychophysiological evidence of anxiety enhancement in ten subjects practicing relaxation.* Paper presented at the Annual Meeting of the Association for the Advancement of Behavior Therapy, New York.

Borkovec, T. D., & Hu, S. (1990). The effect of worry on generalized cardiovascular response to phobic imagery. *Behavior Research and Therapy, 28,* 69–73.

Borkovec, T. D., Lyonfields, J. D., Wiser, S. L., & Diehl, L. (1993). The role of worrisome thinking in the suppression of cardiovascular response to phobic imagery. *Behaviour Research and Therapy, 31,* 321–324.

Borkovec, T. D., & Mathews, A. M. (1988). Treatment of nonphobic anxiety disorders: A comparison of nondirective, cognitive, and coping desensitization therapy. *Journal of Consulting and Clinical Psychology, 56,* 877–884.

Burns, D. D. (1980). *Feeling good: The new mood therapy.* New York: William Morrow.

Clark, D. M. (1994). Cognitive therapy for panic disorder. In B. Wolfe & J. Maser (Eds.), *Treatment of panic disorder: A consensus development conference.* Washington, DC: American Psychiatric Press.

Cioffi, D. (1991). Beyond attentional strategies: A cognitive-perceptual model of somatic interpretation. *Psychological Bulletin, 109,* 25–41.

D'Zurilla, T., & Goldfried, M. (1971). Problem solving and behavior modification. *Journal of Abnormal Psychology, 78,* 107–126.

De Giralamo, G., & McFarlane, A. C. (1996). The epidemiology of PTSD: A comprehensive review of international literature. In A. J. Marsella, M. J. Friedman, E. T. Gerrity, & R. M. Scurfield (Eds.), *Ethnocultural aspects of post-traumatic stress disorder: Issues, research, and clinical applications* (pp. 33–86). Washington, DC: American Psychological Association.

Echebura, E., De Corral, P., Sarasua, B., & Zubrizaretta, I. (1996). Treatment of acute post-traumatic stress disorder in rape victims: An experimental study. *Journal of Anxiety Disorders, 10,* 185–199.

Echebura, E., De Corral, P., Zubrizaretta, I., & Sarasua, B. (1997). Psychological treatment of chronic PTSD in victims of sexual aggression. *Behavior Modification, 21,* 433–456.

Fitzgerald, S. G., & Gonzalez, E. (1994). Dissociative states induced by relaxation training in a PTSD combat veteran: Failure to identify trigger mechanisms. *Journal of Traumatic Stress, 7,* 111–115.

Foa, E. B., Rothbaum, B. O., Riggs, D., & Murdock, T. (1991). Treatment of post-traumatic stress disorder in rape victims: A comparison between cognitive-behavioral procedures and counseling. *Journal of Consulting and Clinical Psychology, 59,* 715–723.

Foa, E. B., Hearst-Ikeda, D. E., & Perry, K. J. (1995). Evaluation of a brief cognitive-behavioral program for the prevention of chronic PTSD in recent assault victims. *Journal of Consulting and Clinical Psychology, 63,* 948–955.

Folkman, S., & Lazarus, R. S. (1980). An analysis of coping in a middle-aged community sample. *Journal of Health and Social Behavior, 21,* 219–239.

Gendlin, E. T. (1996). *Focusing-oriented psychotherapy. A manual of the experiential method.* New York: Guilford Press.

Gleser, G. C., Green, B. L., & Winget, C. (1981). *Prolonged psychosocial effects of disaster: A study of Buffalo Creek.* New York: Academic Press.

Goenjian, A., Najarian, L. M., Pynoos, R. S., Steinberg, A. M., Manoukian, G., Tavosian, A., & Fairbanks, L. A. (1994). Post-traumatic stress disorder in elderly and younger adults after the 1988 earthquake in Armenia. *American Journal of Psychiatry, 151,* 895–901.

Green, B. L., Grace, M. C., & Gleser, G. C. (1985). Identifying survivors at risk: Long-term impairment following the Beverly Hills Supper Club fire. *Journal of Consulting and Clinical Psychology, 53,* 5, 672–678.

Green, B. L., Korol, M., Grace, M. C., Vary, M. G., Leonard, A. C., Gleser, G. C., & Smitson-Cohen, S. (1991). Children and disaster: Age, gender, and parental effects on PTSD symptoms. *Journal of the American Academy of Child and Adolescent Psychiatry, 30,* 945–951.

Green, B. L., Lindy, J. D., Grace, M. C., & Leonard, A. C. (1992). Chronic post-traumatic stress disorder and diagnostic comorbidity in a disaster sample. *Journal of Nervous and Mental Disease, 180,* 760–766.

Herman, J. L. (1992). *Trauma and recovery.* New York: Basic Books.

Horowitz, M. J. (1981). Self-righteous rage and the attribution of blame. *Archives of General Psychiatry, 38,* 1233–1238.

Horowitz, M. J. (1986). *Stress response syndrome* (2nd ed.). Norvale, NJ: Jason Aronson.

Horowitz, M. J. (1993). Stress response syndromes: A review of post-traumatic stress and adjustment disorders. In J. P. Wilson & B. Raphael (Eds.), *International handbook of traumatic stress syndromes* (pp. 49–60). New York: Plenum Press.

Janoff-Bulman, R. (1992). *Shattered assumptions: Towards a new psychology of trauma.* New York: Free Press.

Keane, A., Pickett, M., Jepson, C., McCorkle, R., & Lowery, B. J. (1994). Psychological distress in survivors of residential fires. *Social Science and Medicine, 38,* 1055–1060.

Keane, T. M. (1995). The role of exposure therapy in the psychological treatment of PTSD. *NC-PTSD Clinical Quarterly, 5*(4) 16.

Kubany, E. S., & Manke, F. P. (1995). Cognitive therapy for trauma-related guilt. Conceptual bases and treatment outlines. *Cognitive and Behavioral Practice, 2,* 27-61.

Langer, E. J. (1992). Matters of mind: Mindfulness/mindlessness in perspective. *Consciousness and Cognition, 4,* 289–305.

Lifton, R. J. (1979). The psychology of the survivor and the death imprint. *Psychiatric Annals, 12,* 1011–1020.

Lyons, J. A. (1991). Strategies for assessing the potential for positive adjustment following trauma. *Journal of Traumatic Stress, 4,* 93–111.

Meichenbaum, D., & Fitzpatrick, D. (1993). A constructivist narrative perspective on stress and coping: Stress innoculation application. In L. Goldberger & S. Breznitz (Eds.), *Handbook of stress: Theoretical and clinical aspects.* New York: Free Press.

Myers, D. (1994). *Disaster response and recovery: A handbook for mental health professionals* (DHHS Publication No. (SMA) 94-3010). Washington, DC: U.S. Department of Health and Human Services.

Nezu, A. M., & Carnevale, G. J. (1987). Interpersonal problem solving and coping reactions of Vietnam veterans with post-traumatic stress disorder. *Journal of Abnormal Psychology, 96,* 155–157.

Paulhus, D. L., & Reid, D. (1991). Enhancement and denial in socially desirable responding. *Journal of Personality and Social Psychology, 60,* 307–317.

Pfifer, J. F., & Norris, F. H. (1989). Psychological symptoms in older adults following natural disaster: Nature, timing, duration, and course. *Journal of Gerontology: Social Sciences, 44,* S206–217.

Rando, T. A. (1993). *Treatment of complicated mourning.* Champaign, IL: Research Press.

Resick, P. A., Jordan, C. G., Girelli, S. A., Hutter, C.K. & Marhoefer-Dvorak, S. (1988). A comparative victim study of behavioral group therapy for sexual assault victims. *Behavior Therapy, 19,* 385–401.

Roth, S., & Cohen, L. J. (1986). Approach, avoidance, and coping with stress. *American Psychologist, 41,* 813–819.

Saboonchi, F., & Lundh, L. (1997). Perfectionism, self-consciousness, and anxiety. *Personality and Individual Differences, 22,* 921–928.

Shapiro, E. R. (1994). *Grief as a family process: A developmental approach to clinical practice.* New York: Guilford Press.

Silver, S. M., Brooks, A., & Obenchain, J. (1995). Treatment of Vietnam War veterans with PTSD: A comparison of eye movement desensitization and reprocessing, biofeedback, and relaxation training. *Journal of Traumatic Stress, 8,* 337–342.

Shore, J. H., Tatum, E. L., & Vollmer, W. M. (1986). Psychiatric reactions to disaster: The Mount St. Helens experience. *American Journal of Psychiatry, 143,* 590–595.

Smith, E. M., & North, C. S. (1993).Post-traumatic stress disorder in natural disasters and technological accidents. In J. P. Wilson & B. Raphael (Eds.), *International handbook of traumatic stress syndromes* (pp. 405–419). New York: Plenum Press.

Solomon, Z., Mikulincer, M., & Avitzur, E. (1988). Coping, locus of control, social support, and combat-related post-traumatic stress disorder: A prospective study. *Journal of Personality and Social Psychology, 55,* 279–285.

Solomon, Z., Mikulincer, M., & Flum, H. (1988). Negative life events, coping responses, and combat-related psychopathology: A prospective study. *Journal of Abnormal Psychology, 97,* 302–307.

Tait, R. & Silver, R. C. (1989). Coming to terms with major negative life events. In J. S. Uleman & J. A. Bargh (Eds.), *Unintended thought* (pp. 351–382). New York: Guilford Press.

Taylor, S. E. (1983). Adjustment to threatening events: A theory of cognitive adaptation. *American Psychologist, 38,* 1161–1173.

Taylor, S. E. (1989). *Positive illusions: Creative self-deception and the healthy mind.* New York: Basic Books.

Taylor S. E., & Brown, J. D. (1988). Illusion and well-being: A social-psychological perspective on mental health. *Psychological Bulletin, 103,* 193–210.

Teasdale, J. D., Segal, Z., Willaims, J., & Mark, G. (1995). How does cognitive therapy prevent depressive relapse and why should attentional control (mindfulness) training help? *Behavior Research and Therapy, 33,* 25-29.

Vaughn, K., Armstrong, M. S., Gold, R., O'Conner, N., Jenneke, W., & Tarrier, N. (1994). A trial of eye movement desensitization compared to image habituation training and applied muscle relaxation in post-traumatic stress disorder. *Journal of Behavior Therapy and Experimental Psychiatry, 25,* 283–291.

Vigne, J. (1997). Meditation and mental health. *Indian Journal of Clinical Psychology, 24,* 46–51.

Wahlberg, L. (1997). Selecting patients for trauma focus therapy. *National Center for PTSD Clinical Quarterly, 7,* 1–4.

Watson, C. G., Tuorila, J. R., Vickers, K. S., Gearhart, L. P., & Mendez, C. M. (1997). The efficacies of three relaxation regimens in the treatment of PTSD in Vietnam War veterans. *Journal of Clinical Psychology, 53,* 917–923.

Wenzlaff, R. M., Wegner, D. M., & Roper, D. (1988). Depression and mental control. The resurgence of unwanted negative thoughts. *Journal of Personality and Social Psychology, 55,* 882–892.

Williams, T. (1987). Diagnosis and treatment of survivor guilt. In T. Williams (Ed.), *Post-traumatic stress disorders: A handbook for clinicians* (pp. 75–92). Cincinnati, OH: Disabled American Vets.

Wolfe, J., Keane, T. M., Kaloupek, D. G., Mora, C. A., & Wine, P. (1993). Patterns of positive readjustment in Vietnam combat veterans. *Journal of Traumatic Stress, 6,* 179–193.

Young, B. H. (1992). Traumatic reactivation assessment and treatment: Integrative case examples. *Journal of Traumatic Stress, 5,* 545–555.

Young, B. H. (1990). Facilitating cognitive-emotional congruence in anxiety disorders during self-determined cognitive change: An integrated model. *Journal of Cognitive Psychotherapy: An International Quarterly, 2,* 229–240.

Young, B. H., Drescher, K. D., Kim-Goh, M., Suh, C., & Blake, D. D. (1998). *1992 Los Angeles riot and PTSD: Traumatic exposure and recovery environment factors in Korean-Americans.* Manuscript under editorial review.

Young, B. H., Ford, J. D., Ruzek, J. I., Friedman, M. J., & Gusman, F. D. (1998). *Disaster mental health services: A guidebook for clinicians and administrators.* Menlo Park, CA/White River Junction, VT: National Center for PTSD, Clinical Laboratory & Education/Executive Divisions, Department of Veterans Affairs.

APPENDIX 1. SELF-EXPOSURE TASK RECORD

Name _____   Date _____

Self-Exposure # _____

0 – 10 SUDs RATING

0 = no distress, relaxed
10 = as distressing as being in the traumatic experience itself

Please rate your personal …

Distress at Beginning of Self-Exposure (0-10 rating):   _____

Distress During Self-Exposure (0-10 rating):   _____

Distress After Self-Exposure (0-10 rating):   _____

What Negative Emotions did you have while doing the homework?

1. _____   2. _____   3. _____

What are the new ways of coping with your feelings which you are willing to do now?

1. _____

2 _____

3. _____

4. _____

5. _____

Thanks for filling out this homework form. Remember that by doing self-exposure as part of this group:

•   You'll improve your ability to deal with your memories;
•   You'll learn to handle strong emotions better;
•   You'll begin to break the habit of isolating from others.

NOW, get some support if you need it, and do something active and positive to cope.

APPENDIX 2. LIST OF COPING STRATEGIES

Coping Strategies

Support-Seeking

- Call a friend and ask to talk.
- Get with family and talk.

Relaxation Exercises

- Progressive relaxation.
- Deep breathing.

Time-Out

- Walk away and calm down.

Journal

- Write about the situation and your feelings.

Self-Talk

- Be positive, remind yourself what you've accomplished.
- Be aware of negative distorted thinking.

Regular Exercise

- Walk, swim, bike, stretch, lift weights, etc.

Consistent Daily Routines/Rituals

- Awaken and begin day at same time; eat meals at regularly schedule times; plan recreational or self-care activities that happen daily, weekly or monthly.

Negative Thought Management

- Practice attentional focus and affirmation technique to increase ability to focus and refocus thoughts.

Self-Reward

- Find ways to reward yourself with small gifts, special time, etc.

Distraction through Positive Activities

- Play a sport, go fishing, go to a positive film, etc.

Support Group Attendance

- Go to a meeting.

APPENDIX 3. RECORD OF COPING

Coping with Symptoms

Name _____

Week _____

	Symptom	Situation	Negative Thoughts	Coping Thoughts/Actions
1				
2				
3				
4				

APPENDIX 4. MEMBERS' RELAXATION SKILLS PROGRESS LOG

Relaxation Log

Use this log to measure your progress with the two different self-relaxation techniques. Rate your level of tension/relaxation before and after each practice session using the following scale as a guide:

10	=	Absolutely tense	5	=	Slightly relaxed
9	=	Extremely tense	4	=	Moderately relaxed
8	=	Very tense	3	=	Very relaxed
7	=	Moderately tense	2	=	Extremely relaxed
6	=	Slightly tense	1	=	Absolutely relaxed

$\triangle$ = before
+ = after

Example

10	10	10	10	10	10
9	9	9	9	9	9
8	8	8	8	8	8
7 $\triangle$	7	7	7	7	7
6	6	6	6	6	6
5	5	5	5	5	5
4 +	4	4	4	4	4
3	3	3	3	3	3
2	2	2	2	2	2
1	1	1	1	1	1

5/26/M ____   ____   ____   ____   ____

Date/Technique
Technique: M = muscle; B = breathing;

10	10	10	10	10	10
9	9	9	9	9	9
8	8	8	8	8	8
7	7	7	7	7	7
6	6	6	6	6	6
5	5	5	5	5	5
4	4	4	4	4	4
3	3	3	3	3	3
2	2	2	2	2	2
1	1	1	1	1	1

____   ____   ____   ____   ____   ____

Date/Technique
Technique: M = muscle; B = breathing;

Name: _____

APPENDIX 5. SELF-TALK AND AFFIRMATION TECHNIQUE ASSIGNMENT

Self-Talk Assignment and Affirmation Technique Worksheet

In a recent session we discussed how negative beliefs and distorted interpretations related to your disaster experience may perpetuate distress and impede your recovery. This assignment is designed to help you begin to counter the effects of negative or distorted thinking. Please set time aside to think about the questions listed below before using this worksheet to write down your answers. Bring the completed worksheet to our next session and be prepared to discuss your work. We will help you with any difficulties you might be having with the exercise.

1. After the group's discussion of common negative disaster related thoughts, are you able to identify any such thoughts you have? If yes, please write one or two thoughts down in a sentence.

    Example A: *"My kids will be scarred for life."*

    Example B: *"I was helpless and I'd react that way again."*

Your thought(s): _____

_____

_____

2. Are you willing to view this thought (or these thoughts) as a negative belief or distorted interpretation of your disaster-related experiences that perpetuates your distress?

    Example A: *"Yes, I can see that my being afraid and my concern for my children's welfare has led me to worry excessively about the disaster's impact on them, and that my worrying all the time has got to stop."*

    Example B: *"Yes, I thought I was helpless, but it leaves me feeling unnecessarily worthless because it distorts the fact that I acted in a way that helped me and my family survive."*

_____

_____

_____

Self-Talk and Affirmation Technique Worksheet, p.2

3. Are you willing to believe that you can replace this thought with another thought to counter its negative effect?

    Example A: *"Yes, I can believe that most children are not permanently scarred and can go on to have healthy lives."*

    Example B: *"Yes, I can believe that I am not helpless, and there are countless ways in which I can help myself."*

    _____

    _____

    _____

4. What could you say to yourself to strengthen this counterbelief? Write down three sentences that reflect this counterbelief.

    Example A: 1. *"Children are very resilient and often do well in spite of difficult experiences."*

    2. *"Many children do well in the long run after a disaster."*

    3. *"Giving my children a safe home and lots of love will help them feel secure."*

    Example B: 1. *"I am not helpless."*

    2. *"I help myself all the time."*

    3. *"I can help myself get over what I interpreted as helplessness."*

    _____

    _____

    _____

5. Summarize the three sentences into one sentence.

    Example A: *"My children will be all right with love and support."*

    Example B: *"Helping myself is an act of not being helpless.*

    _____

    _____

Self-Talk and Affirmation Technique Worksheet, p.3

6.   Select from the above sentence, two-to-eight words that represent the sentence's affirmation.

Example A: *"With love and support my children are well."*

Example B: *"I help."*

Please write down your affirmation: _____

_____

_____

7.   Divide this affirmation (phrase) into two or three parts.

Example A:

Part 1: *"With love and support";*   Part 2: *"My children are well."*

Part 1: *"With love";*   Part 2: *"Support";*   Part 3: *"My children are well."*

Example B:

Part 1: *"I";*   Part 2: *"Help."*

_____

_____

8.   Next, practice one of the relaxation techniques you have learned. Immediately afterward (while in a state of relaxation) try repeating the sections of the phrase you wrote down in question 7, selecting Part 1 to focus on during a deep inhalation and Part 2 on a long steady exhalation. If phrase is divided into three parts, the middle part becomes the focus of thought during the two-second holding of breath between inhalation and exhalation. Practice for five minutes several times over the next week and be prepared to discuss your experience at the next session.

Example A:

Inhalation: "With love and support" — *Hold 2 sec.* — *Exhalation: "My children are well."*

Inhalation: "With love" — *Hold 2 sec. "Support"* — *Exhalation: "My children are well."*

Example B:

Inhalation: "I" — *Hold 2 sec* — *Exhalation: "Help."*

Self-Talk and Affirmation Technique Worksheet, p.4

9. Describe an actual situation that would be an opportunity to recall your affirmation.

    Example A: *"My children are misbehaving, and I remind myself that their behavior isn't the result of the earthquake. I remind myself that they are healthy kids who sometimes just misbehave."*

    Example B: *"I am feeling overwhelmed by how much I have to do to restore the house to what it was before the earthquake. I remind myself of how much I have done already and of the fact that I am helping my family return to normalcy."*

    _____

    _____

    _____

    _____

Chapter 10

Group Treatment for Adult Survivors of Childhood Abuse

Lisa Y. Zaidi[1]

PREVALENCE OF CHILDHOOD ABUSE EXPERIENCES

In beginning to address treatment issues for adults abused as children, it is important to first establish the magnitude of the problem. Unfortunately, while many clinicians are keenly aware that the childhood abuse is widespread, a variety of issues impede attempts to accurately assess prevalence (e.g., Williams, 1980). The first problem is definitional. That is, what seems abusive to one individual may not necessarily be so-labeled by another, yielding much variation from study to study (e.g., Baldwin & Oliver, 1975; Helfer & Kempe, 1976). Tied to problems with identifying standardized criteria regarding abusive behavior is a debate about the degree to which various forms of abuse, such as emotional abuse and physical abuse, overlap or coexist. For instance, is sexual abuse a subset, in some sense, of the physically abusive constellation of behaviors? Most researchers and practitioners have addressed these as distinct forms of maltreatment (e.g., Briere, 1992) and yet a cogent case can be made for the view that sexual abuse is by definition a physically abusive act.

A second problem in establishing reliable estimates of prevalence stems from the reluctance of many to report that they have been subjected to childhood maltreatment (Rausch & Knutson, 1991). This may be exacerbated when the abuse has occurred within the context of family and is thus at odds with societal expectations

---

[1] The author would like to gratefully acknowledge the following people for their assistance at various stages of this project: Glenn J. Blumstein, John Briere, Erin Edwards, Fred Gusman, Victoria M. Gutierrez-Kovner, Cheryl B. Lanktree, Judith A. Stewart, my mother Jane K. Zaidi, and the staff at Stuart House in Santa Monica, CA.

regarding the meaning and nature of family. Allen and Bloom (1994) state that "denial of abuse within families—both individual and social—continues to be a major barrier . . . and must be addressed" (p. 431). Thomas, Nelson and Sumners (1994) have eloquently delineated particular impediments to disclosure of sexual abuse of males, which include: (a) expectations that disclosures will reduce their perceived power and efficacy; (b) fears that early experiences or current sexuality, or both, will be labeled as homosexual within the context of a homophobic society; (c) a failure by self and others to define early sexual experiences as abusive versus experimental or forms of sexual initiation; and (d) fears that assumptions will be made regarding their own potential to become abusive.

A third issue, which has waxed and waned in importance during the history of mental health, rests with the willingness of clinicians to acknowledge the widespread nature of childhood maltreatment (Olafson, Corwin, & Summit, 1993). Perhaps beginning with Freud's retraction of the Seduction Theory—that is, his early reports regarding the apparent prevalence of incest in 19th century Vienna—in the wake of vilification and public pressure (Hunt, 1993), our willingness to address child abuse professionally has been tempered by the reaction of the society in which we work and live. The latter half of the century in this country has included renewed awareness and recognition of childhood maltreatment, in many ways beginning with the 1962 publication of *The Battered Child* (Kempe, Silverman, Steele, Droegemiller, & Silver). While many clinicians reluctantly continued to acknowledge the magnitude of the problem, others issued calls for systematic assessment of childhood abuse history as an essential component to be included in any comprehensive mental health assessment (e.g., Briere & Zaidi, 1989; Briere, Lanktree, & Zaidi, 1991; Zaidi & Foy, 1994). Currently, the topic engenders vociferous public reaction and professional factionalization, leading some clinicians to be forced into retreat by threats to their professionalism and accusations that they have peddled the myth of "False Memory." Will history come full circle? Will our understanding that childhood abuse is a vast social problem be replaced by the view that this is a phenomenon manufactured by malicious and incompetent mental health practitioners?

While the three issues cited above have hampered attempts to quantify the prevalence of childhood abuse, several apparently reliable statistics have emerged. Finkelhor, Hotaling, Lewis and Smith (1990) reported that 27% of women and 16% of men experienced childhood sexual abuse. Gelles and Straus (1987) concluded that the rate of severe physical abuse has been approximately 11% to 14% during the past decade. This designation of "severe" distinguishes physical punishment other than spanking, which is apparently normative in the sense that almost all adults report having received some form of physical punishment during childhood (e.g., Knutson & Selner, 1994). Published emotional abuse prevalence rates—the American Humane Association (1981, 1984) reports that between 11%

and 13% of all childhood abuse cases consist of this form of abuse—are viewed as underestimates of the frequency with which this phenomena occurs (e.g., Hart, Germain, & Brassard, 1987). Data show that reports of abuse and neglect have almost tripled since 1980, affecting almost three million children in a single year, and that about half of the reports involve neglect (Children's Defense Fund, 1994). While these statistics are not definitive, they do provide some sense of the magnitude of the problem and establish an imperative for clinicians to address the sequelae of such maltreatment, on both short- and long-term fronts.

EFFECTS OF CHILDHOOD ABUSE EXPERIENCES

Considerable data exist regarding ways in which individuals abused as children may continue to manifest distress during adulthood (e.g., Briere, 1992; Gibson & Hartshorne, 1996; van der Kolk, McFarlane, & Weisaeth, 1996). While a comprehensive review of psychological sequelae is beyond the scope of this chapter, a brief encapsulation of some fundamental themes provides a rationale for particular treatment goals. Long-term psychiatric symptomatology include post-traumatic stress, depression, and anxiety (e.g., Briere, 1992). Self-destructive behaviors, including self-mutilation, substance abuse, suicidality, and eating disorders, are more characteristic of sexual abuse survivors than of members of the general population (e.g., Kreidler & Fluharty, 1994). Childhood coping skills, such as dissociative processes, excessive passivity, and caretaking behaviors, may characterize abused adults (e.g., Kreidler & Fluharty, 1994). Physically abused individuals have been reported to be more aggressive and impulsive than nonabused counterparts (e.g., Friedrich & Wheeler, 1982).

Many investigators have highlighted the impairment of social skills in discussions of long-term effects of childhood abuse. Abused individuals are viewed as less skilled in interpreting social cues and less trusting in interactions (e.g., George & Main, 1979). Allan and Bloom (1994) emphasize this psychological feature as follows:

> No matter which etiologic model is considered, a fundamental aspect of traumatic phenomenology involves disruptions of an individual's relationship with the world. The psychological falling away of an individual from family or society after traumatic exposure is one of the most profound facets of PTSD. (p. 425)

As early as 1947, Newcomb noted that negative attitudes towards others lead to restricted interpersonal communication and contact, thereby preventing any modifications in such attitudes. Perhaps not surprisingly in light of these claims, group treatment has been described as "one of the most effective means of assisting survivors" (Randall, 1995, p. 232). Allan and Bloom stated: "By virtue of their social and interpersonal nature, group . . . therapies provide excellent environments to repair schemas for safety, trust/dependency, independence, power, self-esteem, and intimacy" (1994, p. 426).

Thomas, Nelson, and Sumners (1994) identify five specific ways in which men molested as children can benefit from the group modality. According to these authors, group work has the potential to: (a) reduce isolation; (b) provide opportunities for reality testing; (c) serve as a forum for challenging negative self-beliefs; (d) enable members to identify with and support others; and (e) reduce guilt and shame associated with histories of abuse (p. 104). Although these authors are describing benefits likely to accrue to adult male survivors, there is ample evidence which suggests that female survivors benefit in similar ways (e.g., Sgroi, 1982). In fact, this list of specific potential benefits to adult survivors of abuse is distinctly reminiscent of the curative therapeutic factors identified by theorists of more generic forms of group treatment (Capuzzi & Gross, 1992). What is worth highlighting, however, is that these therapeutic factors, while in many ways characteristic of all effective groups, are perhaps particularly well-suited to the needs of adults abused as children.

While the potential benefits of a group context are clearly tied to particular manifestations of distress, namely social dis-ease, often found in survivors of childhood maltreatment, consideration of other sequelae have the potential to determine the content of the work done within these group contexts.

A THEORETICAL FRAMEWORK

Based on their work with sexually abused children, Browne and Finkelhor (1986) identified four "traumagenic factors" which effectively summarize typical long-term effects of such maltreatment. Although the group model presented in this chapter was not developed solely for survivors of sexual abuse, Browne and Finkelhor's theoretical framework has relevance for the types of difficulties that characterize adult survivors of various forms of maltreatment during childhood. The "traumagenic factors" described by Browne and Finkelhor are:

1 *stigmatization*—impairment of self-concept stemming from feelings of shame, guilt, and perceptions of being "bad" or "damaged";

2 *powerlessness*—general impairment of self-efficacy, particularly in response to perceived authority figures;

3 *betrayal*—diminished sense of trust resulting from the pain and humiliation experienced at the hands of purported caregivers; and

4 *traumagenic sexualization*—inappropriate and dysfunctional sexual behavior of sexual abuse survivors.

For the purpose of the group model described in this chapter, the last factor has been expanded to include difficulties with intimacy and sustained relationships often experienced by victims of various forms of abuse.

Over the years, I have found the framework provided by Browne and Finkelhor's traumagenic factors useful in establishing coherent, relatively holistic, and efficient group treatment protocols. Moreover, Hyde, Bentovim and Monck (1995) recently proposed that building a treatment program around these four traumagenic factors would address the "style and content of treatment" (p. 1396). What follows is a synthesis from 10 years of my work doing just that.

ESTABLISHING THE GROUP: INITIAL CONSIDERATIONS

The group model described in this chapter is intended for adult survivors of childhood maltreatment. This categorization is intentionally broad as discussion of both homogeneous and heterogeneous groups, with respect to abuse histories, is incorporated herein. Depending on the nature of the abuse and limitations imposed by the realities of the treatment setting, I have found it possible to conduct mixed groups comprised of individuals with histories of various forms of maltreatment. This use of mixed groups is at odds with literature which indicates that child abuse groups should be homogeneous (e.g., Blick & Porter, 1982). Certainly group homogeneity is, in many respects, optimal. However, the realities of the settings in which many clinicians work make this not always possible. What does seem therapeutically essential is that each member perceive at least one other member as similar (e.g., Capuzzi & Gross, 1992). Group leaders will also want to avoid any attempts by themselves and by members to evaluate abuse experiences comparatively. Such comparisons distort the subjective reality and undermine the central group goal of destigmatization.

The groups that are the basis for the therapeutic model outlined here were homogeneous with respect to gender. Given the material that tends to emerge around gender role expectations and problems with intimacy, this may actually represent a more fundamental guideline for determining the membership of groups such as these. Mixed gender membership of child abuse groups may pose an insurmountable obstacle for clients already tentative in their willingness to disclose painful material and damaged through their experience of multiple interpersonal failures. If a secondary goal is to facilitate improved relating to members of the opposite sex, the better route may be through mixed gender group leadership. In fact, Black and DeBlassie (1993) argue that such coleadership provides a model of healthy male-female interaction and yields opportunities for acceptance from representatives of both sexes. Other preliminary research data suggests that "a male-female co-counselor team (may) . . . promote . . . the enhancement of self-concept, and the decrease of depression" in a group of female adult survivors of sexual abuse

(Threadcraft & Wilcoxon, 1993, p. 43). Overall, the data suggest that, regardless of gender and whether or not they practice with a cotherapist at all, group counselors must be "caring, nonexploitive, reliable, noncontrolling, and active (Thomas et al., 1994, p. 106)." Ultimately, the primary qualifications are the "knowledge, skills, experience, and personal characteristics" of the counselor working with adult survivors of abuse (Thomas et al., 1994, p. 106).

Another important preliminary consideration rests with the selection of the name for the group. While this might appear trivial, I have not found it to be so. Not surprisingly, potential participants are often leery about joining groups defined by terminology they perceive to be negative. Recalling the research data which indicate that abuse survivors often do not self-label themselves as abused (e.g., Rausch & Knutson, 1991) suggests that potential participants who do not view their experiences as abusive may not even give consideration to joining a group defined in this way. Names such as "Dysfunctional Family Group," "Incest Victims Group," and even "Incest Survivors Group" are viewed negatively by many clients. For instance, adult males sexually abused as children expressed a distinct preference for the designation "males molested as children" (Thomas et al., 1994). Generally, a name such as "Childhood Issues Group" seems less pejorative and, while individual screening of prospective members can establish commonality among members in terms of childhood maltreatment experiences, other members of the community do not necessarily need to know the content of sessions from the group name alone.

As with all groups, considerable thought and effort must precede selection of participants for group treatment (Corey & Corey, 1997). It is useful to create a flyer describing the group in terms of topics to be discussed, fees, qualifications of leaders, duration, frequency and other important information. The flyer should clearly delineate eligibility criteria which, at minimum, includes the following:

1 All participants must have already undergone some individual treatment, they must continue with concurrent individual sessions for the duration of group, and they should plan to continue with individual work upon termination of group.

2 Participants must establish readiness to address childhood abuse issues within a group context.

3 Participants must agree to participate in a pregroup screening interview.

Flyers may be posted, published, and distributed to colleagues in clinical settings.

Once potential members have begun to be identified, group leaders will need to conduct pregroup screening interviews. These interviews are vital to the success of the group (Cole & Barney, 1987) and should be approached as an opportunity for a two-way exchange of information between group leaders and potential participants and a means of mutual determination of whether or not group represents a good fit (Corey & Corey, 1997).

Several important issues need to be considered for the screening interviews. Whenever possible the interviews should be conducted jointly by the coleading pair, with an eye toward modeling effective communication and balance of leadership responsibilities from initial contact with clients. Clients should be given a realistic sense of what the subjective experience of group is likely to be, including the fact that they will "probably feel worse before they feel better"; that others in their interpersonal milieu may not always respond favorably to the changes they may begin to make; and that, despite precautions, there is a potential for inappropriate breaches of confidentiality.

Expectations and limitations of confidentiality, particularly with respect to child abuse reporting laws, must be clarified at the outset. Another issue that often arises with this kind of group work surrounds the nature and degree of communication between group leaders and other professionals involved in treatment. This communication may be particularly thorny in inpatient contexts and further complicated by specific institutional dynamics. For example, many combat veterans with PTSD are wary of implications that their chronic difficulties are traceable to prewar dysfunction, rather than combat trauma. While this is not my position, specific data regarding childhood abuse could potentially be misinterpreted or misused, or both, by other clinical staff or claims adjudicators to support this type of argument.

To address these concerns, I have adopted a stance of informing clients that, while some communication between practitioners is essential, it is neither appropriate nor necessary for details of group disclosures to be shared by group leaders. Rather, leaders will encourage group participants to take the initiative about bringing new and possibly emotionally charged material to the attention of their individual therapists and other members of the treatment team. As a general rule in inpatient settings, it is sufficient for most staff members to simply know that participants are involved in work related to childhood abuse. Adjunct staff on inpatient units and members of a treatment team will appreciate, however, if attempts are made to inform them that a given member may, for example, have had a hard time in group today.

Another example of appropriate sharing of information would be for a group facilitator to alert the individual therapist that a client disclosed additional material regarding, for instance, childhood abuse history which may be important to process on a one-on-one basis. This should be done without revealing the exact nature of the group-specific disclosure if at all possible. The individual therapist can then

approach the client as follows: "I understand that something else about your childhood came up in group today and that you were upset. Would you like to talk about
it now with me?" Approaching sensitive material in this way preserves the integrity of the group experience while still enabling a group facilitator to, in a sense,
collaborate with his or her colleagues.

When working with adult survivors of abuse it is essential to be vigilant against
inadvertent and tactless sharing of material processed during group sessions. The
essence of effective group work is trust. A powerful way to establish trust is to
delineate the parameters of interstaff communication for clients and fellow professionals at the outset of the group.

Other issues discussed during the screening interview include commitment to
the group, outpatient follow-up, and group structure and expectations. Guidelines
regarding the content and purpose of the screening interviews are consistent with
established procedures identified by group theorists such as Corey and Corey (1997)
and do not need to be restated here. Following the interview, the leaders and potential members are given a week to assess whether the purpose of the group is compatible with individual needs. Those who elect not to participate or who are ex-
cluded by the leaders are provided with more appropriate referrals. Qualified individuals electing to participate are asked to complete a written contract to remain in
the group for the preestablished duration.

GROUP STRUCTURE

The group model described herein entails a relatively short-term treatment approach. Clearly a short-term framework is more consonant with current trends in
psychotherapy but, in the case of work with adult survivors of childhood abuse, it
may actually be optimal from a clinical standpoint as well. For instance, Herman
and Schatzow (1984) have cogently argued that a time-limited approach facilitates
rapid bonding and diminishes resistance to sharing emotionally loaded material.
In addition, it provides a structure which contains the intensity and modulates the
often disorganizing and regressive aspect of abuse-focused treatment.

Like everything else, short-term is a relative designation and will be, to some
extent, dictated by the specific therapeutic context (e.g., inpatient versus outpatient) and other factors, such as staffing and funding considerations. Time frames
for the childhood abuse groups described herein ranged from five weeks of twice
weekly 90-minute sessions for inpatients on a PTSD unit receiving multiple forms
of concurrent treatment to three months of weekly hour-long meetings for outpatient groups. The treatment model outlined can be adjusted to accommodate various short-term time frames through expansion or reduction of time devoted to the
various treatment modules.

The group process is sequentially structured to address specific treatment goals as follows:

1 develop cohesiveness and build initial trust;

2 incorporate a psychoeducational component regarding child abuse;

3 explore family of origin dynamics;

4 process memories of childhood maltreatment on affective and cognitive levels;

5 facilitate appropriate expression of anger;

6 examine obstacles to intimacy;

7 promote awareness of disciplinary options and explore parenting dilemmas; and

8 begin to plan for the future.

Selection of these topics is rooted in Browne and Finkelhor's traumagenic factors model (1986) and in clinical experience with adult survivors. However, it now appears that the topics are also consistent with a study of "curative factor rankings" by female incest survivors (Randall, 1995). Randall summarized three studies and found the most important therapeutic factors to be: cohesiveness, self-understanding, and family reenactment. Catharsis was also important for participants in short-term groups and seemed to be "linked to early group members' attempts to gain relief" (Randall, 1995, p.235). Thus, we see an overlap between theoretical conceptualizations, clinical perspectives, and the expressed treatment needs of clients.

Treatment Goal 1: Building Group Cohesiveness

Establishing cohesiveness and fostering trust are essential precursors to detailed discussions of childhood abuse experiences. A variety of introductory activities are useful in promoting bonding and establishing the environment in which painful material can be shared. Rather than asking members to introduce themselves, they can be asked to pair up and "interview" one another before presenting information about each other to the group. Depending on the group, members can be asked to choose partners or randomly assigned a partner. I often use puzzle halves from a children's game which members draw from a hat. They then have to circulate and find the person holding the matching half. This eliminates anxiety surrounding whether or not members will be chosen and adds a degree of levity to this initial activity.

Following these introductions, members are given a preliminary group outline which they are asked to modify by rank-ordering topics and suggesting alternative issues to be addressed. This road map appears to reduce anxiety and enhance participants' sense of control over the group process.

Next, a variety of warm-up exercises can be useful for expanding the behavioral repertoire of group members. I often use preliminary art exercises suggested by Naitove (1988). First, clients are given three sheets of blank paper. Then they are asked to "put whatever (they) would like on the page" and given 10 seconds to do this for each paper. Next clients are asked to go back and provide a title for each page. Finally, they share the pages with the group. Ostensibly, the squiggles provide information regarding unconscious material, whereas the naming is more rooted in conscious processes. The real utility of the activity, however, lies in its ability to free clients from constricted behavior patterns. Clients are often surprised by the time constraints for this activity and may want to process reactions to being unable to "complete" an ambiguous task.

Often in tandem with the squiggle activity, I ask clients to complete an "Aspects of Life" drawing in which they fill a page with drawings or words, or both, relating to seven areas of their lives as follows: Me, Family, Anger, Joy, Work, Play, Love. Another useful art exercise entails asking clients to draw the way they are feeling right now (Capacchione, 1989). This last activity is one that I also encourage clients to complete on their own between sessions and to share with the group at their discretion.

Participants may also be asked to complete a self-drawing and drawing of a member of the opposite sex. These drawings, which are a variant of the House-Tree-Person test (Buck, 1948; Klepsch & Logie, 1982; Koppitz, 1968) are used to explore self-concepts, including body image, and affect, as well as perceptions of members of the opposite sex. Although such drawings can be used for diagnostic purposes and have been used as pre- and postgroup assessment measures (e.g., Gutierrez-Kovner, Zaidi, & Lanktree, 1990), my preference is that group members interpret their own artwork. Thus, art was viewed as a supplement to verbal communication and as a window on potentially relevant clinical material while avoiding the powerlessness sometimes engendered by limiting expression regarding a piece of art to therapist interpretations.

A variety of drama therapy exercises can also provide a means of physically warming up for group (e.g., Emunuh, 1994). While many exercises can be helpful, one that I often employ was developed by Naitove (1988) in order to enhance physical awareness, provide opportunities for nonverbal communication, and discharge initial anxiety. For this exercise, members form a circle and follow the therapists around the room, pretending to walk through mud, across ice, through leaves, etc. Next, they engage in Body Writing, where they stand in a circle facing each other and "write" their names in the air with their nose, left and right index fingers, elbows, and left and right big toes. They write their names in large and small letters and then turn outward to write with their backsides. Typically, this last part of the activity induces humor and reduces tension in the room.

Other activities used to promote cohesiveness include having members jointly develop group rules and group goals, which I then photocopy and disseminate to the group. Group cohesiveness and group identity are further fostered by establishing a predictable routine for sessions. Meetings begin and end by "checking in" with members since powerful feelings, and perhaps new memories, often surface between and during group meetings. Whenever possible, snacks and coffee are provided as clients convene before the session and are brought into the therapy room during the "check in" process. This is consistent with Blick and Porter's (1982) recommendations that the "symbolic nurturance" provided through the sharing of refreshments may be particularly important for survivors of childhood maltreatment.

The main activity scheduled for each session occurs after these introductory activities. At the end of each session members are apprised of upcoming changes in routine and prepared for the topic of the following session, and feedback and suggestions are solicited from participants. Finally, each meeting ends with a "checking in" which has as a focus the members' current emotional status and reflections on what transpired in group that day. To maximize the therapeutic benefit of this time-limited treatment approach, group members are requested to complete exercises between sessions and encouraged to collect thoughts and drawings in a journal to be shared at their discretion. Several good workbooks provide guidelines for appropriate journal exercises (e.g., Capacchione, 1989; Cohen, Barnes, & Rankin, 1995; Davis, 1990).

Other activities that are useful during the initial stage of group development include asking participants to bring to group an object that is in some way representative of them. I prefer to have this happen quickly, preferably during the second meeting. Members are asked to refrain from sharing their objects before group (otherwise they will often share them in the waiting room before group begins) and to plan to say something about what this object represents about them. This activity is illuminating for the sharing member and observers alike. It sets the stage for trust and allows members to begin to self-disclose. Participants will choose to define themselves in a variety of ways, not exclusively tied to their abusive experiences.

In a similar vein, I often ask clients to complete Self-Collages, which they bring to an early meeting, perhaps the third. They are instructed to complete a collage which represents who they are and to describe it to the group during the next meeting. Since participants will have varying degrees of access to craft materials, group leaders choosing to use this activity may need to be prepared to provide materials such as poster board, magazines, scissors, and glue. As with the Personal Objects, this exercise promotes sharing and also begins the process of disclosing personal material. In addition, both activities enable members to discern ways in which they are similar beyond having experienced maltreatment during childhood. Group leaders can facilitate this bonding process by highlighting similarities and common interests of members. All of this relates to the ultimate goal of destigmatizing abused clients and enabling them to feel less isolated and damaged by their experiences.

Treatment Goal 2: Education About Child Abuse

An early presentation, preferably during the first group meeting, of psychoeducational material including descriptions of various forms of abuse and prevalence rates is also intended to address the stigmatization associated with a history of abuse. Specific intentions are to reinforce that all members of the group have been harmed in some way during childhood, to mitigate self-blame (Cole, 1985), and to lay the groundwork for reframing survivor behaviors as constructive adaptations to adversity. Typically, this material is presented using a handout which members can take with them.

Treatment Goal 3: Sharing the Family Context

Once the group is launched and a basis for authentic communication has been established through completion of some of the above exercises, members are instructed to complete simple genograms which they then share with the group (Kerr & Bowen, 1988). Genograms are used to diagram the quality of primary relationships within the family of origin and to provide a basis for discussion of cultural backgrounds, family roles, expectations, and cross-generational patterns. Describing their family provides an opportunity for each group member to explore family dynamics and establishes a context for abusive experiences disclosed during the course of the group. For example, in describing his family, one group member began to cry as he shared feelings of being acutely alone because, unlike the others, he no longer had contact with any of his family following abandonment by them at age 12. Apparently, viewing a schematic representation of his family, which was mostly a blank page, allowed intense feelings of loss and isolation to surface and was more eloquent than a raft of words.

Treatment Goal 4: Confronting Memories of Abuse

Prior to sharing their abusive histories, members are asked to complete a Time Line of key childhood experiences. This exercise is used to facilitate disclosure of specific abusive events, which begins as soon as possible after the above treatment goals have been met, potentially during the fourth or fifth sessions. Sharing abuse histories early in the group process minimizes stigmatization, eliminates secrecy surrounding abusive incidents, and reduces the anticipatory anxiety associated with waiting to disclose what actually happened.

Members take turns detailing their abusive childhood histories over the span of approximately three group meetings. This segment of the group is less structured and is planned to enable ample processing of abusive incidents, cathartic affective expression, cognitive reworking of the events, and examination of adaptive and maladaptive survivor behavioral patterns.

A useful strategy, proposed by Kreidler and Fluharty (1994), involves including a processing session after every three or four stories in order to address leaders' and members' feelings of being "overwhelmed by the continued intensity of the disclosure phase" (p. 177). Specific issues to be addressed at this time include: "commonalties of feelings, trigger points, fears, symptoms (which usually increase at this time), nightmares, flashbacks, and difficulties within the group process and with group members. . . . Safety mechanisms are stressed" (pp. 177-178).

In an attempt to expand their repertoire of coping skills, group members are given basic instruction in relaxation techniques using a graduated approach beginning with deep breathing, followed by progressive muscle relaxation, and, finally, guided imagery (e.g., Goldfried & Davison, 1976). These techniques are presented as potentially useful coping measures rather than universally effective means of reducing anxiety since relaxation exercises may actually intensify feelings of powerlessness and, hence, paradoxically, increase rather than decrease subjective levels of anxiety among survivors of childhood abuse (Briere, 1989).

Following disclosure of their abusive histories, members are asked to write a letter to an abused child. This exercise, completed between sessions, is used to access empathic feelings for the child within and to heighten awareness that a child is never culpable for abuse perpetrated against him or her (Davis, 1990). Members read their letters aloud during a subsequent session and the group explores the myriad emotions stirred in writer and listeners alike.

Treatment Goal 5: Expressing the Anger

A similar letter-writing exercise involves composing a letter to an abuser. These letters, written to explore often avoided feelings of anger (Davis, 1990), are also shared with the group. Subsequent discussion enables members to ventilate pent up rage in a directed and nonviolent manner. One group participant had such difficulty forming words to express his anger that his first attempt to write led to stabbing the page with a pen and then crumpling the paper in frustration. Later, he was able to sit down and, for the first time in his life, give voice to the tremendous pain and anger that stemmed from his molestation.

The two letters described above and several other written exercises given as homework between sessions are derived from the *Courage to Heal Workbook* (Davis, 1990). Other exercises drawn from this source and assigned intermittently throughout the remainder of the group focus on:

- learning to attend to the inner voice that directs responses to various situations;

- developing awareness of messages internalized from childhood and how such messages affect self-concept as well as perceptions of how one is viewed by others; and

- attending to thoughts and attitudes about sex.

Group members are also provided with written information regarding typical cognitive distortions (e.g., Burns, 1980) and are encouraged to attend to such distortions in their own and other members' perceptions of events.

Treatment Goal 6: Exploring Obstacles to Intimacy

The art therapy technique of collage can be effectively used to explore group participants' thoughts and feelings regarding a variety of issues, such as perceptions of the self and of others and views about roles in their families of origin (e.g., Gutierrez-Kovner et al., 1990). A particularly powerful use of collage is as a vehicle for discussion of male-female relationships. For this activity, participants are given poster board, scissors, glue, and a wide variety of magazines during a session, perhaps the eighth meeting. They are instructed to divide the poster in half, write "MEN" on one side and "WOMEN" on the other and affix photographs or words, or both, reflecting their conception of "what it means to be a man" and "what it means to be a woman" under each heading. The collages are completed during the first part of the session and then shared with other participants. During the process of sharing, members are asked to describe underlying themes of their collage as well as to indicate the basis for selection of each individual component. Unlike the Self-Collages, these collages are completed individually during group time so as to access free associative material, relatively uncontaminated by elaborate cognitive processes and psychological defenses.

These collages, which convey a lot of information regarding sex roles, provide a basis for discussion of intimacy, sexuality, and relationships. Specifically, sharing the collages enables members to explore perceptions that may have interfered with their ability to form lasting, intimate relationships with desired partners. Over the years, interesting patterns have emerged. For instance, most members of one male survivor group depicted females as happy, attractive, and carefree, whereas males were represented as solemn, angry, and burdened by the troubles of the world. Photographs selected for the male sides of some of the collages included a prisoner in shackles, coal miners, soldiers, and infamous dictators. One individual's collage summarized this theme by including a smiling theatrical mask on top of the female side and a frowning mask on top of the male side. The similarity between the three collages was striking since all participants completed the project independently. Themes which have emerged with female survivor groups have centered around the sexualization of women and men as aggressors. In one instance, a female survivor included a painting of a cowering caged woman which she surrounded by images of men in business suits.

Treatment Goal 7: Learning About Effective Discipline

Given evidence suggestive of multigenerational transmission of parenting styles (Zaidi, Knutson, & Mehm, 1989), one session toward the end of the treatment sequence includes a psychoeducational presentation of effective disciplinary tactics. Group members are given handouts describing a rationale for discipline versus punishment and are instructed in basic behavioral parenting principles as well as specific techniques, such as "time out." This information, presented and detailed in a written how-to format, provides the basis for group discussion and problem-solving. Members are given another handout which summarizes appropriate developmental expectations for children of different ages. In addition, group members participate in role-play exercises designed to improve communication with their children by decreasing the ambiguity of commands, and clarifying the connection between failure to comply and specific consequences. Although not all group members are parents, it is believed that most have or will have access to children and will have occasion to draw upon information regarding parenting not based on their own childhood experiences.

Treatment Goal 8: Planning for the Future

Termination is anticipated and discussed in a graduated manner as the final date approaches. Members are encouraged to explore feelings related to the ending of group and to examine ways in which their current reactions mirror personal responses to other losses or endings in their lives. Members and leaders engage in assessment of what has been learned and the identification of high and low points, as well as turning points, in the group process. In an attempt to consolidate learning and generalize to the world outside of group, members identify issues requiring further exploration, anticipate potential challenges and obstacles, and discuss plans for follow-up treatment.

The final meeting ends with appropriate rituals, often of the members' choosing. These may include the designation of a Magic Box filled with material that members wish to leave behind as they exit the group (Emunuh, 1994). Other groups have chosen to establish a final page in their journals as a place for autographs from other members, which are completed during the last part of the final meeting. Members sometimes elect to take group photographs or exchange addresses and telephone numbers so as to maintain contact after group ends. I like to distribute diplomas, symbolic of the achievement of the end of group and the commencement of a new phase. Finally, group ends with the sharing of refreshments—often a cake—and a celebration of the courage inherent in members' willingness to confront painful childhood memories.

CONCLUSION

Patten, Gatz, Jones, and Thomas (1989) have articulated the goal of treatment for survivors of childhood abuse as "recovery from trauma (which) occurs when a victim is transformed into a survivor who is able to integrate the catastrophe into his or her life history and use it as a source of strength" (p. 198). The group treatment protocol described in this chapter is intended to be implemented with this overarching goal in mind.

On more concrete levels, this group model represents an effort to address systematically specific identified sequelae of childhood abuse, including post-traumatic stress symptomatology, through an amalgam of treatment techniques. Evidence suggests that treatment for survivors of childhood abuse must "recognize the unique needs of adult survivors, avoid strict adherence to any single theory, and create a plan that incorporates a variety of strategies" (Thomas et al., 1994, p. 108). The present treatment model incorporates psychoeducational, cognitive, behavioral, psychodynamic, and expressive arts therapy elements. The time frame outlined for this group model, which presents a deliberate sequenced order for topics to be addressed, is intentionally conducive to modification based on leader preference and institutional constraints. While the model is a time-limited one, individual treatment components may be expanded or reduced to suit the needs of a particular group. One caveat to this flexibility is that leaders should preestablish the duration of their particular group whenever possible so as to minimize ambiguity and associated member anxiety.

Although this group treatment is eclectic and flexible, it is grounded in the conceptual framework provided by the work of Browne and Finkelhor (1986). Specifically, fostering a nurturing, predictable, and safe therapeutic environment, where each member is treated with dignity and respect, counters expectations of betrayal. Consistent with this goal, the confidentiality of detailed disclosures is maintained unless legal or safety concerns dictate otherwise. Participation in a group comprised of other individuals with similar histories reduces feelings of stigmatization. Early sharing of abusive experiences minimizes members' feelings of shame surrounding the abuse, prevents protracted speculation about what might have happened to others, and reduces anticipation about telling their story. Feelings of powerlessness stemming from childhood victimization by adults, which is analogous to the learned helplessness that characterizes humans and animals repeatedly exposed to uncontrollable maltreatment (Seligman, 1974), is addressed in several ways:

- by empowering group members to make decisions about group rules, confidentiality, and topics to be discussed;

- by enabling individuals to determine how much they are ready to share at a given time; and

- by encouraging the creator to interpret his or her own artwork by "guiding" exploration of the work rather than providing an interpretation.

In addition, group members learn parenting techniques which enable them to feel effective during stressful encounters with children. Traumagenic sexualization (Browne & Finkelhor, 1986) and problems with intimacy and sustained relationships are addressed through cognitive exercises, artwork, and group discussion.

Developmental considerations dictate the need to utilize modalities other than the verbal therapies for the exploration of feelings and memories associated with a history of childhood abuse. For this reason, art therapy techniques such as those described above are viewed as fundamental to therapists treating the sequelae of abuse (Jacobson, 1991; Naitove, 1982, 1988). Although adults will often demonstrate initial resistance about art therapy and drama therapy exercises, which are typically outside their zone of comfort, I have found these methods invaluable in fostering flexibility, encouraging spontaneity, and helping clients identify alternative, nonverbal means of expressing themselves. Early responses may include those similar to one expressed by one of my former clients, a burly ex-convict who stood well over six feet tall and announced when given craft materials during the first group meeting, "I ain't gonna carry around no crayons." Ultimately, he relented and, like the other members, came to appreciate the utility of these nonverbal techniques.

Despite the breadth and complexity of the treatment goals identified in this chapter, several studies reveal that childhood abuse survivors asked to evaluate their own group experiences most value the curative factors of cohesiveness and self-understanding (e.g., Randall, 1995). This suggests that group leaders specializing in treatment of adult survivors should not lose sight of foundational principles of group dynamics. In particular, time and effort devoted to pregroup planning, screening interviews, and the early trust-building phase of group development represent the therapeutic building blocks upon which positive treatment outcome depends.

REFERENCES

Allen, S. N., & Bloom, S. L. (1994). Group and family treatment of post-traumatic stress disorder. *Psychiatric Clinics of North America, 17,* 425–437.

American Humane Association. (1981). *National study on child neglect and reporting.* Denver: Author.

American Humane Association. (1984). *National study on child neglect and reporting.* Denver: Author.

Baldwin, J. A., & Oliver, J. E. (1975). Epidemiology and family characteristics of severely abused children. *British Journal of Preventative and Social Medicine, 29,* 205–221.

Berger, A. M., Knutson, J. F., Mehm, J. G., & Perkins, K. A. (1988). The self-report of punitive child experiences of young adults and adolescents. *Child Abuse and Neglect, 12,* 251–262.

Black, C. A., & DeBlassie, R. R. (1993). *Adults molested as children: A survivor's guide for women and men.* Orwell, VT: Safer Society Press.

Blick, L. C., & Porter, F. S. (1982). Group therapy with female adolescent incest victims. In S. M. Sgroi (Ed.), *Handbook of clinical intervention in child sexual abuse* (pp. 147–175). Lexington, MA: DC Heath.

Briere, J. (1989). *Therapy for adults molested as children: Beyond survival.* New York: Springer Publishing.

Briere, J. (1992). *Child abuse trauma: Theory and treatment of the lasting effects.* Newbury Park, CA: Sage Publications.

Briere, J., & Zaidi, L. Y. (1989). Sexual abuse histories and sequelae in female psychiatric emergency room patients, *American Journal of Psychiatry, 146,* 1602–1606.

Browne, A., & Finkelhor, D. (1986). Initial and long-term effects: A conceptual framework. In D. Finkelhor (Ed.), *A sourcebook on child sexual abuse* (pp. 180–198). Beverly Hills, CA: Sage Publications.

Buck, J. N. (1948). The house-tree-person technique: A qualitative scoring manual. *Journal of Clinical Psychology, 4,* 317–396.

Burns, D. D. (1980). *Feeling good: The new mood therapy.* New York: Signet.

Capacchione, L. (1989). *The creative journal: The art of finding yourself.* North Hollywood, CA: Newcastle Publishing.

Capuzzi, D., & Gross, D. R. (1992). *Introduction to group counseling.* Denver: Love Publishing.

Children's Defense Fund. (1994). *The state of America's children.* Washington, DC: Author.

Cohen, B. M., Barnes, M., & Rankin, A. B. (1995). *Managing traumatic stress through art: Drawing from the center.* Lutherville, MD: The Sidran Press.

Cole, C. H., & Barney, E. E. (1987). Safeguards and the therapeutic window: A group treatment strategy for adult incest survivors. *American Journal of Orthopsychiatry, 57,* 601–609.

Cole, C. L. (1985). A group design for adult female survivors of childhood incest. *Women and Therapy, 4,* 71–82.

Corey, M. S., & Corey, G. (1997). *Groups: Process and practice.* Pacific Grove, CA: Brooks/Cole.

Davis, L. (1990). *The courage to heal workbook: For women and men survivors of child sexual abuse.* New York: Harper & Row.

Emunuh, R. (1994). *Drama therapy: Process, technique, and performance.* New York: Brunner/ Mazel.

Finkelhor, D., Hotaling, G., Lewis, I. A., & Smith, C. (1990). Sexual abuse in a national survey of adult men and women: Prevalence, characteristics, and risk factors. *Child Abuse and Neglect, 14,* 19–28.

Friedrich, W. N., Berliner, L., Urquiza, A. J., & Beilke, R. L. (1988). Brief diagnostic group treatment of sexually abused boys. *Journal of Interpersonal Violence, 3,* 331–343.

Friedrich, W. N., & Wheeler, K. K. (1982). The abusing parent revisited: A decade of psychological research. *The Journal of Nervous and Mental Disease, 170,* 577–587.

Gelles, R. J., & Straus, M. A. (1987). Is violence toward children increasing? A comparison on 1975 and 1985 national survey rates. *Journal of Interpersonal Violence, 2,* 212–222.

George, C., & Main, M. (1979). Social interactions of young abused children: Approach, avoidance and aggression. *Child Development, 50,* 306–318.

Gibson, R. L., & Hartshorne, T. S. (1996). Childhood sexual abuse and adult loneliness and network orientation. *Child Abuse and Neglect, 20,* 1087–1093.

Goldfried, M. R., & Davison, G. C. (1976). *Clinical behavior therapy.* New York: Holt, Rinehart, & Winston.

Gutierrez-Kovner, V. M., Zaidi, L. Y., & Lanktree, C. B. (1990, April). *Group treatment with sexually abused latency-aged girls.* Paper presented at the Seventh Biennial Meeting of the National Symposium on Child Victimization, Atlanta.

Hart, S. N., Germain, R., & Brassard, M. R. (1987). The challenge: To better understand and combat the psychological maltreatment of children and youth. In M. R. Brassard, R. Germain, & S. N. Hart (Eds.), *Psychological maltreatment of children and youth* (pp. 3–24). New York: Pergamon.

Helfer, R. E., & Kempe, C. H. (1976). *Child abuse and neglect: The family and the community.* Cambridge, MA: Ballinger.

Herman, J., & Schatzow, E. (1984). Time-limited group therapy for women with a history of incest. *International Journal of Group Psychotherapy, 34,* 605–616.

Hunt, M. (1993). *The story of psychology.* New York: Anchor Books.

Hyde, C., Bentovim, A., & Monck, E. (1995). Some clinical and methodological implications of a treatment outcome study of sexually abused children. *Child Abuse and Neglect, 19,* 1387–1399.

Jacobson, M. (1991, June). *Art therapy with survivors of childhood abuse.* Paper presented at the Eastern Regional Conference on Child Abuse and Multiple Personality Disorder, Arlington, VA.

Kempe, C., Silverman, F., Steele, B. Droegemueller, W., & Silver, H. (1962). The battered-child syndrome. *Journal of the American Medical Association, 181,* 17–24.

Kerr, M. E., & Bowen, M. (1988). *Family evaluation.* New York: Norton.

Klepsch, M., & Logie, L. (1982). *Children draw and tell: An introduction to the projective uses of human figure drawings.* New York: Brunner/Mazel.

Knutson, J. F., & Selner, M. B. (1994). Punitive childhood experiences reported by young adults over a 10-year period. *Child Abuse and Neglect, 18,* 155–166.

Koppitz, E. M. (1968). *Psychological evaluation of children's human figure drawings.* New York: Grune & Stratton.

Kreidler, M. C., & Fluharty, L. B. (1994). The "new family" model: The evolution of group treatment for adult survivors of childhood sexual abuse. *The Journal for Specialists in Group Work, 19,* 175–181.

Naitove, C. E. (1982). Art therapy with sexually abused children. In S. M. Sgroi (Ed.), *Handbook of clinical intervention in child sexual abuse* (pp. 269–308). Lexington, MA: DC Heath.

Naitove, C. E. (1988, April). *Art therapy treatment techniques for abused children.* Workshop conducted at the Sixth Biennial Meeting of the National Symposium on Child Victimization, Anaheim, CA.

Newcomb, T. (1947). Autistic hostility and social reality. *Human Relations, 1,* 69–86.

Olafson, E., Corwin, D. L., & Summit, R. C. (1993). Modern history of child sexual abuse awareness: Cycles of discovery and suppression. *Child Abuse and Neglect, 17,* 7–24.

Patten, S., Gatz, Y., Jones, B., & Thomas, D. (1989). Post-traumatic stress disorder and the treatment of sexual abuse. *Social Work, 34,* 197–203.

Powell, L. P., & Faherty, S. L. (1990). Treating sexually abused latency age girls: A 20-session plan utilizing group process and the creative arts therapies. *The Arts in Psychotherapy, 17,* 35–47.

Randall, D. A. (1995). Curative factor rankings for female incest survivor groups: A summary of three studies. *The Journal for Specialists in Group Work, 20,* 232–239.

Rausch, K., & Knutson, J. F. (1991). The self-report of personal punitive childhood experiences and those of siblings. *Child Abuse and Neglect, 15,* 29–36.

Seligman, M. E. (1974). *Learned helplessness.* San Francisco: Freeman Press.

Sgroi, S. M. (1982). *Handbook of clinical intervention in child sexual abuse.* Lexington, MA: DC Heath.

Thomas, M. C., Nelson, C. S., & Sumners, C. M. (1994). From victims to victors: Group process as the path to recovery for males molested as children. *The Journal for Specialists in Group Work, 19,* 102–111.

Threadcraft, H. L., & Wilcoxon, S. A. (1993). Mixed-gender group co-leadership in group counseling with female adult survivors of child sexual victimization. *Journal for Specialists in Group Work, 18,* 40–44.

van der Kolk, B. A., McFarlane, A. C., & Weisaeth, L. (Eds.). (1996). *Traumatic stress: The effects of overwhelming experience on mind, body, and society.* New York: Guilford.

Williams, G. J. (1980). Child abuse and neglect: Problems of definition and incidence. In C. J. Williams & J. Money (Eds.), *Traumatic abuse and neglect of children at home.* Baltimore, MD: Johns Hopkins University Press.

Zaidi, L. Y. (1994). Group treatment of adult male inpatients abused as children. *Journal of Traumatic Stress, 7,* 719–727.

Zaidi, L. Y., & Foy, D. W. (1994). Childhood abuse experiences and combat-related PTSD. *Journal of Traumatic Stress, 7,* 33–42.

Zaidi, L. Y., & Gutierrez-Kovner, V. M. (1992). Group treatment of sexually abused latency-age girls. *Journal of Interpersonal Violence, 10,* 215–227.

Zaidi, L. Y., Knutson, J. F., & Mehm, J. G. (1989). Transgenerational patterns of abusive parenting: Analog and clinical tests. *Aggressive Behavior, 15,* 137–152.

Afterword

Trauma survivors who develop PTSD face many difficult challenges. Many of these challenges present themselves in social and interpersonal domains as the survivors struggle to cope with stigmatization and feelings of alienation, inadequacy, guilt, helplessness, and rage. Group therapy provides a therapeutic community wherein the survivor can process these reactions. In addition, the group setting provides a safe environment to process the trauma, receive and give support, and observe and practice new methods of coping. From a societal view, group therapy is valuable also because of its cost-efficiency. One or two therapists can deliver treatment simultaneously to numerous trauma survivors.

The preceding chapters comprise what is arguably the most succinct and informed summary currently available on group therapy for trauma survivors. The timeliness of their publication cannot be overstated. About 20 years have elapsed since the formal recognition of trauma as an etiological factor in psychiatric disorder (American Psychiatric Association, 1980). Despite the exponential growth of PTSD literature in that time, little has been published to guide practitioners or scientists on how to conduct and examine this mainstay modality for trauma therapy. This book signals a new era aimed at substantiating and empirically verifying the efficacy of group therapy for trauma survivors, as well as providing a snapshot of where the field currently stands.

The dawning millenium offers an opportunity to review critically the state of the art of Group Therapy with trauma survivors. First, and perhaps foremost, it is readily apparent that the application of group therapy to trauma survivors is woefully understudied. Methodologically rigorous research, employing credible control conditions and using random assignment, is needed to examine group therapy for PTSD in general and as it differentially applies to particular trauma populations. In this regard, several issues call for study. First, identifying which type of group treatment works best for what type of patient (i.e., patient-treatment matching) is extremely important and will be immediately valuable to the practitioner. For example, the relative advantages of here and now problem-oriented, process-oriented treatments, and treatments that are exposure-based or entail some form of trauma focus or revivification, should be examined. Second, traditional group therapy issues such as optimal group size, open versus closed formats, time-limited versus open-ended formats, didactic versus process modalities, confrontational versus supportive approaches, and other issues are also important for study.

When to deliver treatment is another important factor to study, as is amply apparent in PTSD, where many acute trauma patients spontaneously remit or regain favorable adjustment. Along these lines, it is important to study the so-called adjusted (or resilient) trauma survivors; indeed, most survivors adjust well and return to their pretrauma levels of functioning. The behavior and experiences of well-adjusted survivors provide important clues about what constitutes therapeutic (or recovery) factors that can be implemented via group therapy (e.g., fostering trust, providing unconditional support), and what it should address (e.g., psychological issues of safety, loss, or intimacy). How much group therapy is optimal is also important to assess. Is more group therapy better therapy? The answer to this question is not clear. Greater amounts of group treatment may not in practice lead to commensurate gain, as appears true for inpatient PTSD treatment (Fontana & Rosenheck, 1997). Finally, the role that the therapist should adopt—a highly active role, as in the case of psychoeducation, cognitive therapy, and exposure based therapy, or a relatively passive-observational one, as in the case of milieu- and process-oriented groups—is also important to examine, not only for PTSD treatment but for group therapy as a whole.

Group therapy may be essential for treating large numbers of trauma survivors, such as those surviving natural disasters, car accidents, and rape. Furthermore, as suggested by the chapters contained in this volume, group therapy may be the treatment of choice for trauma survivors. Potentially, no other treatment modality equals group therapy's capability to attenuate the emotional, cognitive, and behavioral effects of exposure to pervasive trauma. Although the expense and energy involved in providing group treatment to the many people exposed to trauma may be considerable, the costs of not taking that step may be far greater. Group therapy interventions may provide at least a partial remedy to this need.

We note with great excitement the growing public interest in the psychological consequences of trauma exposure. Still, widespread public denial of the impact of tragedy is a reality that survivors and helpers contend with on a continual basis. Listening to the accounts and feelings of people who have been tortured, abused, or horrified, can increase our own sense of vulnerability and helplessness, and challenge our faith in justice and humanity. Many choose to believe that wars, rapes, incest, accidents, and disasters leave no emotional scar, insisting that, while these phenomena are tragic, they and their effects are distant and temporary. The facts, however, indicate otherwise. Trauma is pervasive, and it often leaves an enduring legacy of fear, anxiety, anger, and emotional pain.

Widespread human suffering challenges any society or culture to maintain its empathic and abiding faith in humanity. It challenges each of us to reaffirm our relatedness, compassion, and caring for one another. People who are cognizant of the psychological effects of trauma exposure and how these effects are best offset, e.g., by providing social and emotional support, arranging group debriefings and opportunities for reprocessing, will not only support efforts to help survivors outside the therapy setting, but may better prepare people to seek treatment when they experience trauma. In this case, a better informed public is a more prepared and responsive public. We hope this book helps to bring us closer toward that end.

B.H.Y.

D.D.B.

REFERENCES

American Psychiatric Association. (1980). *Diagnostic and statistical manual of mental disorders* (3d ed.). Washington, DC: Author.

Fontana, A., & Rosenheck, R. A. (1997). Effectiveness and cost of the inpatient treatment of post-traumatic stress disorder: Comparison of three models of treatment. *American Journal of Psychiatry, 154,* 758–765.

Index

comorbid alcohol abuse, 121–123
disaster workers, 66–67
disaster-related groups, 163–164
military veterans, 82–83
sexual assault survivors, 38–39, 47
Scurfield, R. M., 70, 77–79, 81
Secondary gain, 95–96
Secondary traumatization, 21, 54
families, 20–21
sexual assault survivors, 41, 48
Seduction theory (Freud), 202
Segal, Z., 156
Self-care, 5–8, 80
Self-cohesion, 6, 8
Self-defeating behaviors
child abuse survivors, 203
military veterans, 84–85, 87
Self-disclosure, 7–8
Self-esteem, 6
disaster survivors, 154
disaster workers, 35, 39–40, 45–46
military veterans, 77, 84, 86
Self-exposure task, 182–183, 193
Self-management skills training, 128–130,
151, 156–162, 167–175
Self-medication, 119
Self-mutilation, 39
Seligman, M. E., 217
Selner, M. B., 202
Separation distress, 139–141
groups, 144–146
Sexual assault survivors, 3, 7, 35–50, 137, 222
children, 201–220
contraindications, 47–48
empirical research, 36–38
military veterans, 92–95
techniques, 38–47
therapist's role, 46–47
Sexual dysfunction, 35
Sgroi, S. M., 204
Shalev, A., 61
Shame, 9
child abuse survivors, 204
disaster survivors, 152
family approach, 20
military veterans, 78, 80–81, 85, 91, 97
Shapiro, E. R., 163
Shatan, C. F., 75
Shatzow, 1
Shaw, S. R., 120
Shelton, R. B., 32
Sher, K., 119, 121

Shoham, S., 62, 76
Shopshire, M. S., 88
Shore, J. H., 149
Silberman, E. K., 58
Silver, H., 202
Silver, R. C., 154, 156
Silver, R. L., 69
Silver, S., 77
Silverman, F., 202
Singer, M. T., 16
Sison, G.F.P., 107
Skleber, 4
Sleep disturbance
comorbid alcohol abuse, 125–126
military veterans, 89
Sleep hygiene, 126
Smith, C., 202
Smith, E. M., 57, 149
Social Adjustment Scale, 3
Social phobias, 123
Social skills training, 130–132
Social support
comorbid alcohol abuse, 131–132
disaster survivors, 151
Solomon, S. D., 57, 62, 76
Solomon, Z., 157
Sonnega, 101
Sorensen, D. J., 88
Southwick, S. M., 83, 121
Spencer, H., 118
Spielberger, C. D., 108
Spitznagel, E. L., 118
Spouse involvement
accident survivors, 112
disaster workers, 61–62
Spungen, D., 137
Stages by Dimensions Model, 2, 5–8, 13
Stages of Recovery (Herman), 7
Standardized Assault Interview, 3
State-Trait Anxiety Inventory, 3, 108
Steele, B., 202
Steinmetz, J., 113
Stewart, J. A., 89, 93–95, 201
Stewart, S. H., 118–119
Stigmatization, 204
Stiver, I. P., 18, 25
Stratakis, C. A., 53
Straus, M. A., 202
Stress Inoculation Training, 35–37, 112
Stress management, 8
disaster survivors, 152
disaster workers, 52–54

Veterans' Administration, 76, 83, 86, 93
  Vet Centers, 75–76, 93, 118, 123, 128
Vickers, K. S., 156
Victims of Violence Program, 2, 5, 7–9
Vietnam Veteran Counseling Services, 75–76
Vietnam war, 76–97, 118–119
Vigne, J., 156
Virgil, 85
Vollmer, W. M., 149

W

Wagner, B. M., 17
Wahlberg, L., 163
Wakefield, K., 96
Walker, J. I., 76, 88
Walsh, W., 35
Ward, C. H., 39, 108
Watson, C. G., 156
Watzlawick, P., 16
Weathers, F. W., 107–108
Wegner, D. M., 157
Weisaeth, L., 56, 203
Weiss, D. S., 78, 89
Weiss, R. D., 120
Weissberg, M. P., 54
Wenzlaff, R. M., 157
West, J. A., 89
Wheeler, K. K., 203
Wilcoxon, S. A., 206
Williams, G. J., 201
Williams, J., 156
Williams, T., 187
Wilmer, N., 108
Wilson, G. T., 130
Wilson, J. P., 96
Windle, M., 119

Wine, P., 157
Winnicott, 80–81
Winston, T., 67
Wiser, S. L., 156
Wisniewski, N., 35
Withdrawal, 20, 67
Wolfe, J., 117, 157
Wolpe, J., 102–103
Women Veterans' Health Clinics, 93
Women
  military veterans, 91–95
  therapists, 96–97
Women's Health Affairs (VA), 93
Women's Health Sciences Division (VA), 93
Women's Stress Disorder Treatment programs
  (VA), 93
Women's Trauma Recovery Program, 93
Women's War Memorial, 95
Woods, M., 77
World War II, 75–76, 87, 102
Wortman, C. B., 69
Writing activities, 40–42, 46, 76, 109–111,
  194, 213
Wynne, L. C., 16

Y ~ Z

Yalom model, 3
Yalom, I. D., 18
Yehuda, R., 83
Young, B., 149–150, 156, 163, 167, 172
Zahn-Waxler, C., 18
Zaidi, J. K., 201
Zaidi, L. Y., 202, 210, 215
Zimering, R. T., 106, 132
Zubizarreta, I., 156
Zucker, R. A., 15